Muscular Dystrophies

Edited by Kunihiro Sakuma

Published in London, United Kingdom

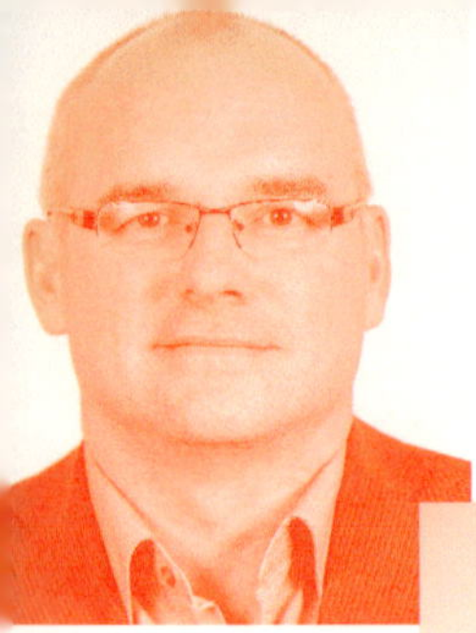
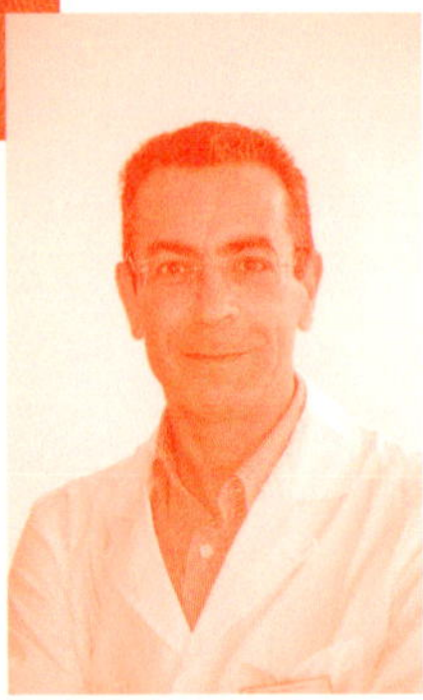
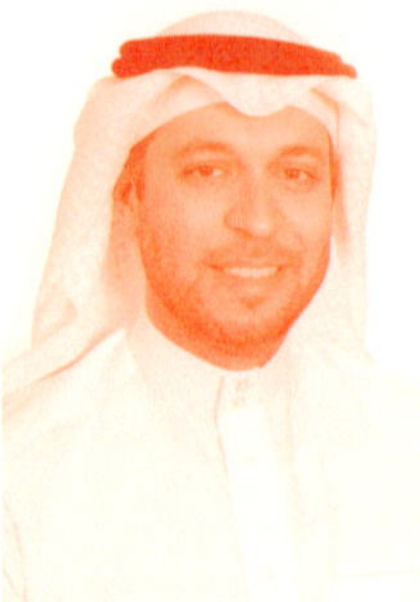
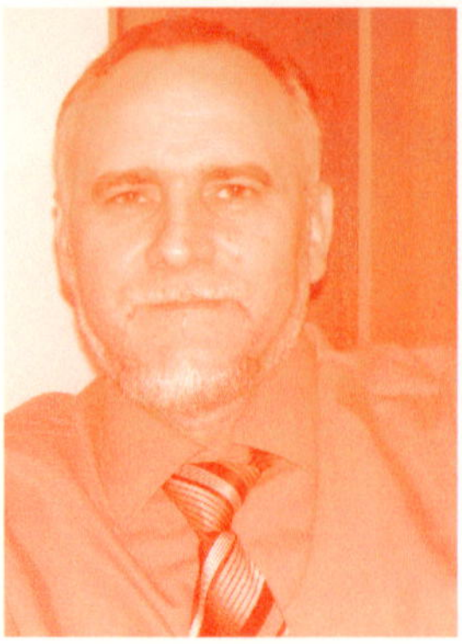
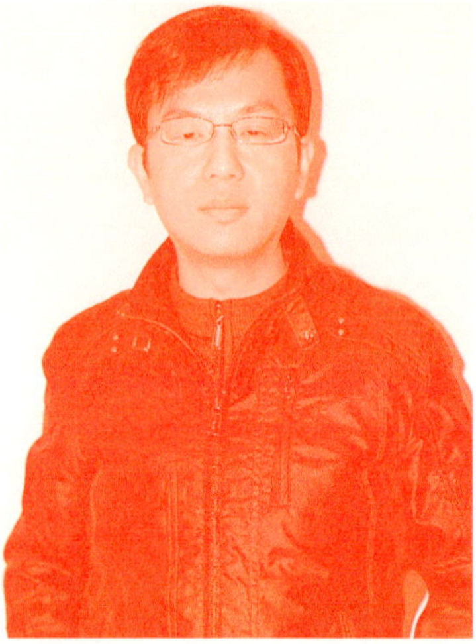
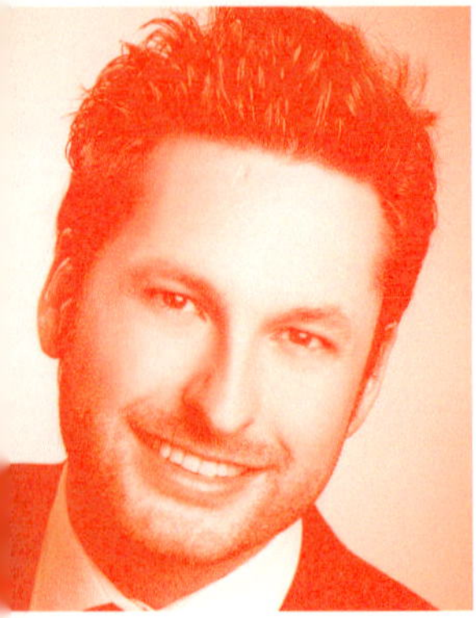
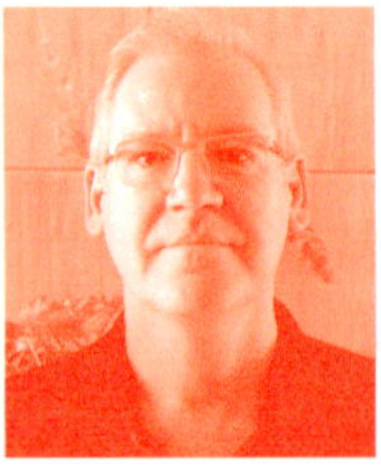

IntechOpen

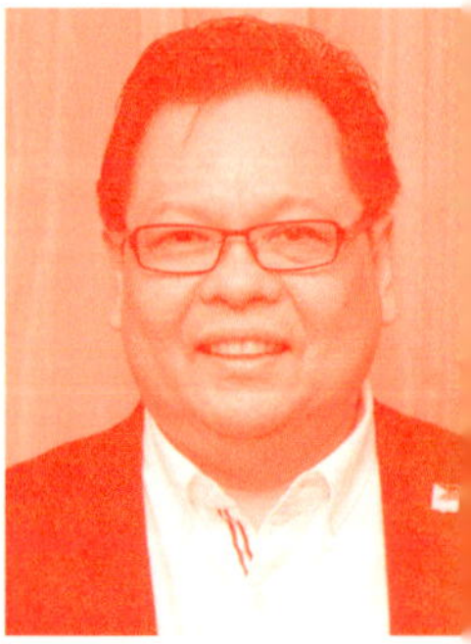
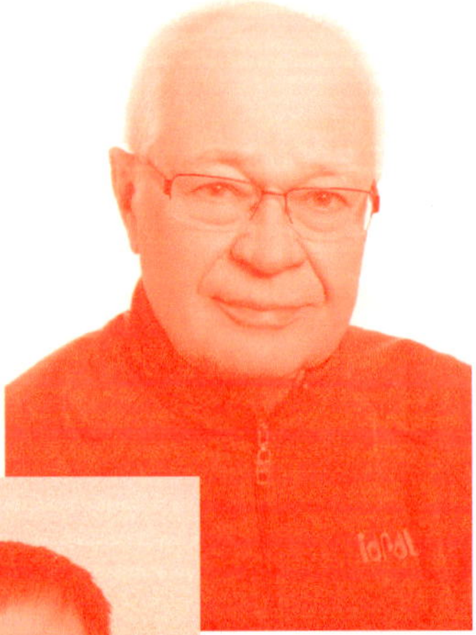
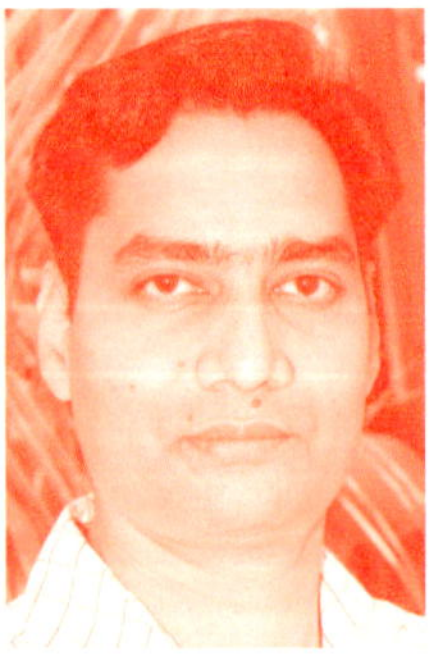
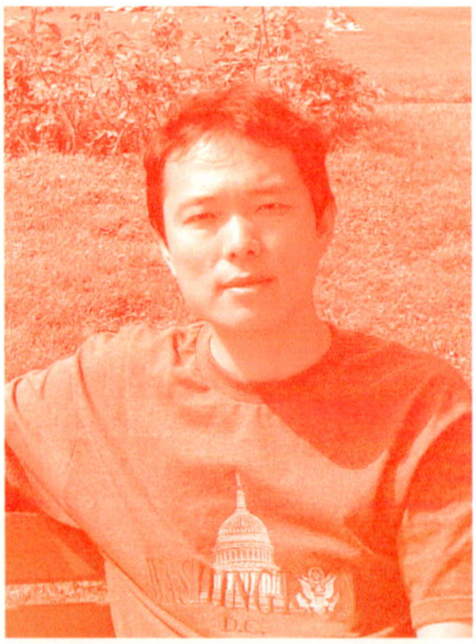
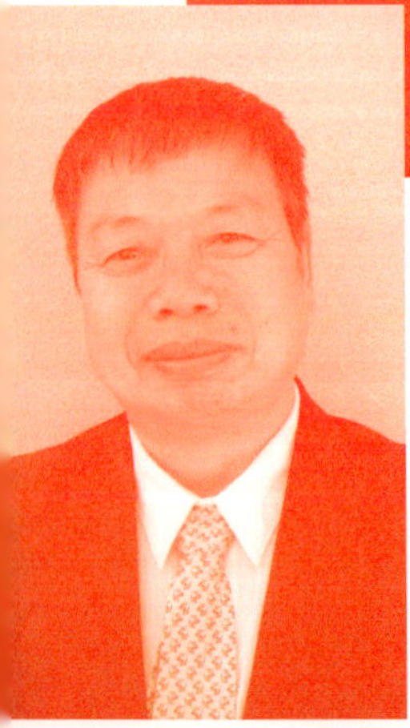
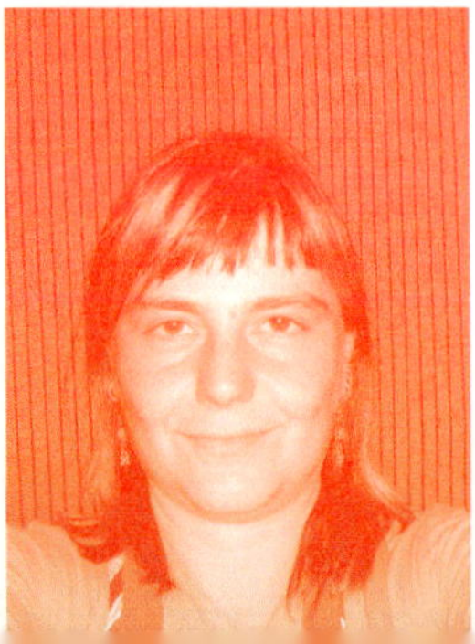

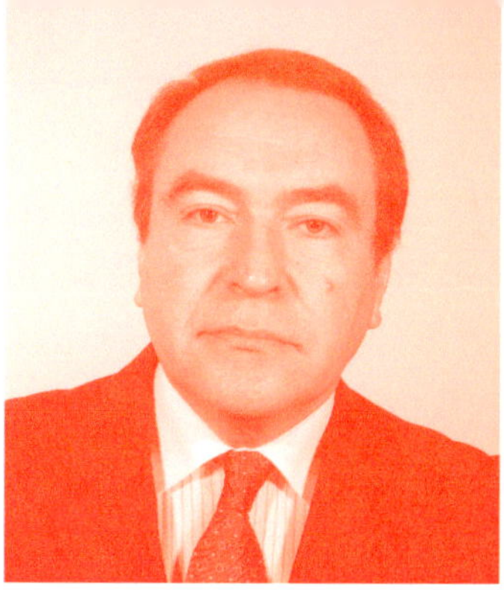
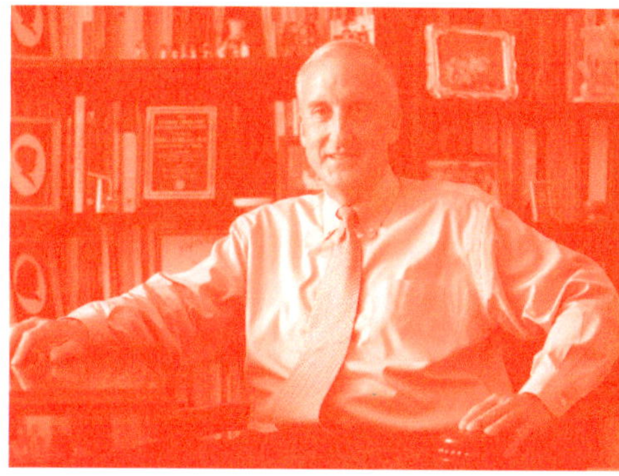
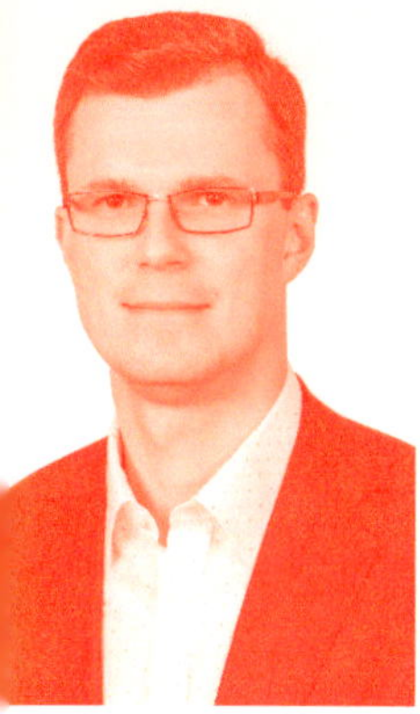
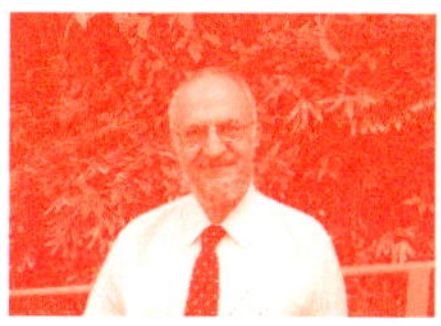
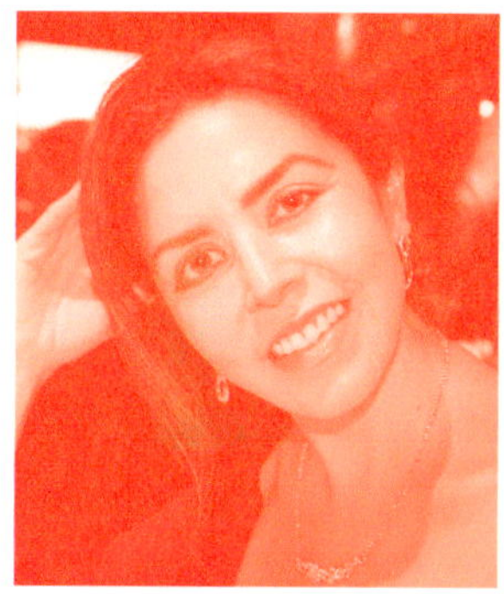

Supporting open minds since 2005

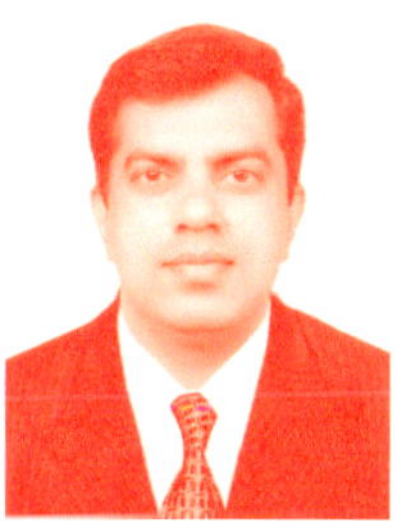
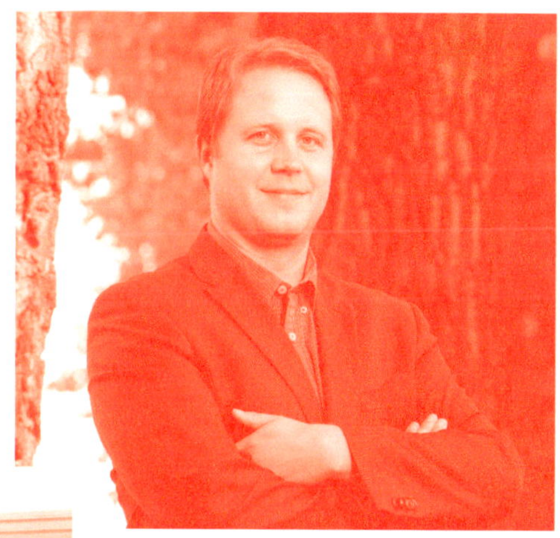
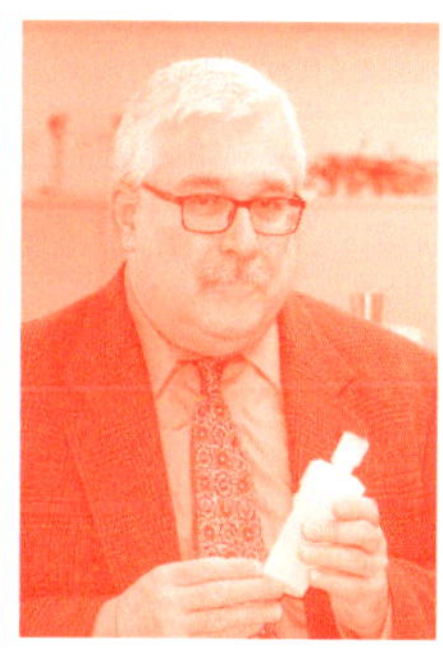
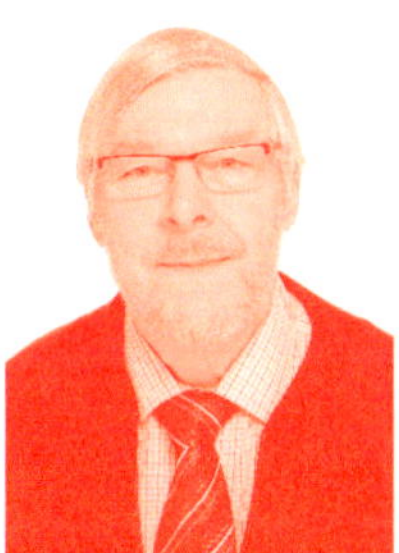
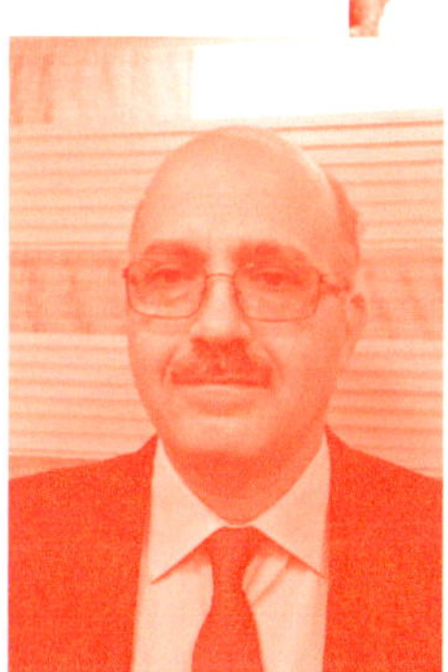
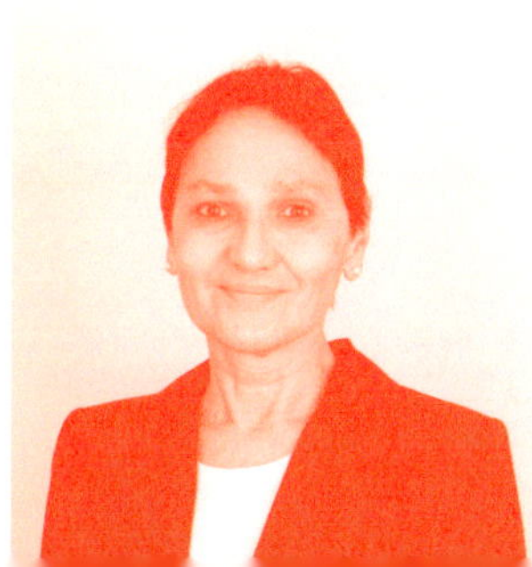
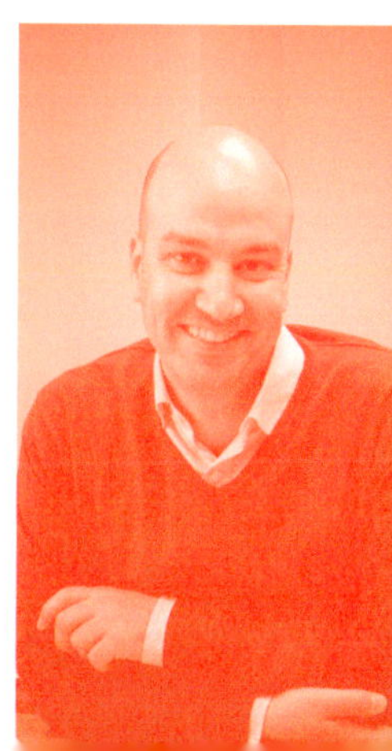

Muscular Dystrophies
http://dx.doi.org/10.5772/intechopen.73974
Edited by Kunihiro Sakuma

Contributors
Gisela Gaina, Magdalena Budisteanu, Elena Ionica, Emilia Manole, Tomoko Yamamoto, Yoichiro Kato, Noriyuki Shibata, Sally Lloyd, Roger Dawkins, Jose Valenzuela, Francis Mastaglia, Yukihiko Ueda, Fabio Iannotti, Samuel Honório, Marco Batista, João Serrano, Helena Mesquita, João Petrica, Jorge Santos, Júlio Martins, Jaime Ribeiro, Stefan Golaszewski, Kunihiro Sakuma

First published in London, United Kingdom, 2019 by IntechOpen
IntechOpen is the global imprint of INTECHOPEN LIMITED, registered in England and Wales, registration number: 11086078, The Shard, 25th floor, 32 London Bridge Street
London, SE19SG - United Kingdom
Printed in Croatia

British Library Cataloguing-in-Publication Data
A catalogue record for this book is available from the British Library

Additional hard and PDF copies can be obtained from orders@intechopen.com

Muscular Dystrophies
Edited by Kunihiro Sakuma
p. cm.
Print ISBN 978-1-78923-845-7
Online ISBN 978-1-78923-846-4
eBook (PDF) ISBN 978-1-83962-224-3

For EU product safety concerns:
IN TECH d.o.o., Prolaz Marije Krucifikse Kozulić 3, 51000 Rijeka, Croatia, info@intechopen.com or visit our website at intechopen.com.

Meet the editor

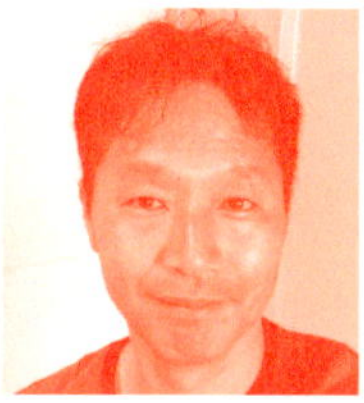

Professor Kunihiro Sakuma, PhD, currently works at the Institute for Liberal Arts at the Tokyo Institute of Technology. He is a physiologist working in the field of skeletal muscle. He was awarded a sports science diploma in 1995 by the University of Tsukuba and started scientific work at the Department of Physiology, Aichi Human Service Center, focusing on the molecular mechanism of congenital muscular dystrophy and normal muscle regeneration. His interest later turned to the molecular mechanism and attenuating strategy of sarcopenia (age-related muscle atrophy). His ambition is to attenuate sarcopenia by improving autophagic defects using nutrient- and pharmaceutical-based treatments.

Contents

Preface

Skeletal muscle is a highly plastic organ that is modulated by various pathways controlling protein turnover. Loss of muscle is a serious consequence of many chronic diseases and of aging. Muscle loss is also common in muscular dystrophy, in which marked loss of various proteins such as the dystrophin–glycoprotein complex occurs around muscle fibers. The autophagy-dependent system and ubiquitin–proteasome signaling (UPS) are well known as major intracellular degradation systems, and their appropriate function is crucial to health and muscle homeostasis. Indeed, muscle wasting and weakness such as cachexia, dystrophy, and sarcopenia is characterized by marked decreases in protein content, muscle fiber size, and muscle strength. The apparent defect of autophagy-dependent signaling is observed in various muscular dystrophies. The adaptive changes of UPS are highly controversial in Duchenne muscular dystrophy (DMD), limb-girdle muscular dystrophy, and Ullrich congenital muscular dystrophy.

Many researchers have investigated exercise-based, supplemental, pharmacological, gene therapy approaches to attenuate various muscular dystrophies. Currently, there is no cure for patients suffering from muscular dystrophies. Although several researchers actively try to determine the effect of pharmacological inhibition of myostatin for DMD patients, it is very difficult for obtaining positive effects and there are few possibilities of its clinical application. Glucocorticoids (GCs) are commonly used and still serve as a gold standard therapy. Nowadays, weekly, intermittent GC treatment has been shown to provide a better alternative to a daily regimen. More recently, attention has been paid to induced pluripotent stem cell technology and its potential application in DMD treatment, although almost all studies use DMD model mdx mice. In addition, the strategy using CRISPR/Cas9 technology progressed dramatically for the restoration of functional dystrophin. An increasing number of studies report successful and beneficial effects of CRISPR/Cas9 only animal models of muscular dystrophy. Thus, it seems necessary that genome editing tools be applied the dystrophic patients for some time to come.

This book provides a comprehensive overview of the various muscular dystrophies, including characteristics, diagnosis, and classification. General treatment of drugs (e.g. corticosteroids) and physical therapy for muscular dystrophies are discussed. In addition, current applications for cell and tissue engineering using muscle stem cells or gene therapy are introduced. This book also deals with the recent advances in appropriate models of drug screening using cell cultures or mammalian organs in vitro in this field.

Kunihiro Sakuma
Professor
Tokyo Institute of Technology,
Tokyo, Japan

Section 1

Introduction

Chapter 1

Introductory Chapter: Muscular Dystrophy and Recent Therapeutic Strategy

Kunihiro Sakuma

1. Introduction

Skeletal muscle tissue accounts for almost half of the human body mass. Human health is markedly affected by any deterioration in the material, metabolic, and contractile properties of skeletal muscle. Skeletal muscle is a highly plastic organ that is modulated by various pathways controlling cell and protein turnover.

Loss of muscle is a serious consequence of many chronic diseases and of aging itself. Muscle loss is also common in muscular dystrophy, in which marked loss of various membranous structural proteins occurs around muscle fibers [1]. Defects in components of the dystrophin-glycoprotein complex (DGC) are known to be an important cause of different muscular dystrophy.

Nowadays, the autophagy-dependent system and ubiquitin-proteasome signaling (UPS) are well known as a major intracellular degradation system, and its appropriate function is crucial to health and muscle homeostasis. Indeed, muscle wasting and weakness such as cachexia, dystrophy, and sarcopenia is characterized by marked decreases in the protein content, muscle fiber size, and muscle strength. Interestingly, a functional defect in autophagy-dependent signaling in sarcopenic mice and humans was recently suggested [2, 3]. In addition, apparent defect of autophagy-dependent signaling is also observed in various muscular dystrophies. Indeed, De Palma et al. [4] have described marked defect of autophagy in dystrophin-deficient mdx mice and Duchenne muscular dystrophy (DMD) patients through the electron microscopic evaluation of muscle tissue and decreased autophagic regulator proteins (i.e., Bnip3, Atg12, and LC3-II). The adaptive changes of UPS are highly controversial in several muscular dystrophies such as DMD, LGMD, and Ullrich congenital muscular dystrophy [5], although UPS seems to not be activated in human sarcopenic muscle [6].

2. Various therapeutic approaches for muscle dystrophy

To attenuate various forms of muscular dystrophy, many researchers have investigated exercise-based, supplemental, pharmacological, and gene therapy approaches. Currently, there is no cure for patients suffering from muscular dystrophies. Although several researchers actively try to determine the effect of pharmacological inhibition of myostatin for DMD patients, it is heavily difficult to obtain positive effects and there are few possibilities for clinical application. Indeed, a randomized clinical trial of anti-myostatin for DMD patients had a trend toward improved muscle mass and performance, but was stopped early due to non-muscle

IntechOpen

side effects (i.e., epistaxis and telangiectasias) [7]. Glucocorticoids (GCs) are commonly used and still serve as a gold standard therapy, acting as anti-inflammatory drugs [8]. More recently, weekly, intermittent GCs treatment has been shown to provide a better alternative to a daily regimen without eliciting muscle atrophy [9]. Recently, more attention is paid to induced pluripotent stem cells (iPSCs) technology and their potential application in DMD treatment [10], although almost all studies used DMD model mdx mice. In addition, the strategy using CRISPR/Cas9 technology progressed dramatically for the restoration of functional dystrophin [11]. Young et al. [12] have found that removal of exons 45–55 resulted in the expression of the stable dystrophin protein in both cardiomyocytes and skeletal myotube in vitro. An increasing number of studies report successful and beneficial effects of CRISPR/Cas9 only animal models of muscular dystrophy. Thus, it seems to be necessary for substantial time for genome editing tools to apply the dystrophic patients.

Author details

Kunihiro Sakuma
Institute for Liberal Arts, Environment and Society, Tokyo Institute of Technology, Tokyo, Japan

*Address all correspondence to: sakuma@ila.titech.ac.jp

References

[1] Vainzof M, Ayub-Guerrieri D, Onofre PC, Martins PC, Lopes VF, Zilberztajn D, et al. Animal models for genetic neuromuscular disease. Journal of Molecular Neuroscience. 2008;**34**(3):241-248

[2] Carnio S, LoVerso F, Baraibar MA, Longa E, Khan MM, Maffei M, et al. Autophagy impairment in muscle induces neuromuscular junction degeneration and precocious aging. Cell Reports. 2014;**8**(5):1509-1521

[3] Sakuma K, Kinoshita M, Ito Y, Aizawa M, Aoi W, Yamaguchi A. p62/SQSTM1 but not LC3 is accumulated in sarcopenic muscle of mice. Journal of Cachexia, Sarcopenia and Muscle. 2016;7(2):204-212

[4] De Palma C, Morisi F, Cheli S, Pambianco S, Cappello V, Vezzoli M, et al. Autophagy as a new therapeutic target in Duchenne muscular dystrophy. Cell Death & Disease. 2012;**3**:e418

[5] Sakuma K, Aoi W, Yamaguchi A. The intriguing regulators of muscle mass in sarcopenia and muscular dystrophy. Frontiers in Aging Neuroscience. 2013;**6**:230

[6] Sakuma K, Aoi W, Yamaguchi A. Molecular mechanism of sarcopenia and cachexia: Recent research advances. Pflügers Archiv/European Journal of Physiology. 2017;**469**(5-6):573-591

[7] Campbell C, McMillan HJ, Mah JK, Tarnopolsky M, Selby K, McClure T, et al. Myostatin inhibitor ACE-031 treatment of ambulatory boys with Duchenne muscular dystrophy: Results of a randomized, placebo-controlled clinical trial. Muscle & Nerve. 2017;**55**(4):458-464

[8] Ciafaloni E, Moxley RT. Treatment options for Duchenne muscular dystrophy. Current Treatment Options in Neurology. 2008;**10**(2):86-93

[9] Quattrocelli M, Barefield DY, Warner JL, Vo AH, Hadhazy M, Earley JU, et al. Intermittent glucocorticoid steroid dosing ehnahces muscle repair without eliciting muscle atrophy. Journal of Clinical Investigation. 2017;**127**(6):2418-2432

[10] Kalra S, Montanaro F, Denning C. Can human pluripotent stem cell-derived cardiomyocytes advances understanding of muscular sydtrophies? Journal of Neuromuscular Diseases. 2016;**3**(3):309-332

[11] Salmaninejad A, Valilou SF, Bayat H, Ebadi N, Daraei A, Yousefi M, et al. Duchenne muscular dystrophy: An updated review of common available therapies. The International Journal of Neuroscience. 2018;**128**(9):854-864

[12] Young CS, Hicks MR, Ermolova NV, Nakano H, Jan M, Younesi S, et al. A single CRISPR-Cas9 deletion strategy that targets the majority of DMD patients restores dystrophin function in hipsC-derived muscle cells. Cell Stem Cell. 2016;**18**(4):533-540

Section 2

The Diagnosis of Muscular Dystrophy

Chapter 2

Clinical and Molecular Diagnosis in Muscular Dystrophies

Gisela Gaina, Magdalena Budisteanu, Emilia Manole and Elena Ionica

Abstract

Muscular dystrophies are a diverse group of inherited muscle disorders with a wide range of clinical manifestations from a severe form with early onset and early death to adult forms with later onset and minimal clinical manifestation that do not affect life-span. Overlapping clinical symptoms and the multitude of genes that need to be analyzed for an accurate characterization make the diagnosis hard. In next-generation sequencing era, a lot of used assay in molecular diagnostics must be taken into consideration for muscular dystrophy diagnosis. However, for more accurate diagnosis, muscle protein expressions analysis may have prognostic value. In this chapter, we present the most important clinical and laboratory findings in the most common forms of muscular dystrophies and molecular diagnostic approaches for a more accurate diagnosis.

Keywords: muscular dystrophy, multiplex Western blot, immunofluorescence, MLPA, hrMCA, dystrophin, calpain 3, *DMD* gene, CAPN3, genetic diagnosis

1. Introduction

Muscular dystrophies (MD) are an inherited group of genetic disorders clinically characterized by progressive muscular weakness and wasting [1] and reduced skeletal muscle mass until their destruction due to a primary defect in the muscle cell. To date, there are known more than 30 different forms of MD with specific signs, symptoms, and genetic basis but sharing common histological features like variation in fiber shape and size and the presence of degeneration and regenerating fibers and connective tissue proliferation [2]. The diseases are distinguished from one another by the age of onset, muscles affected, as well as rate of disease progression [3]. While for some forms of MD, the initial symptoms manifested begin with childhood and have a rapid progression of muscle weakness causing the death of the patients around the age of 20 years, the other forms debut later in adulthood [4, 5] and have a slow rate of progression and an almost normal lifetime [6, 7]. Also, heart disease and mental retardation accompany some types of MD [8, 9], suggesting a different pathogenesis of the disease. It also found that there are subtypes of MD that share similar clinical manifestations and different genetic defects with similar clinical manifestation [10, 11].

However, the progress made in the past 33 years, since the first protein involved in a type of muscular dystrophy was discovered, leads to identify a large number of the genes as well as novel proteins involved in these muscle disorders [12].

For a rapid and an accurate diagnosis improvement in analysis, methods have become a necessity. The combination of clinical signs with muscle histopathology

IntechOpen

and protein and genetic analyses becomes the diagnostic gold standard for these disorders. Nevertheless, for many patients with yet unidentified muscular dystrophy, the diagnosis continues to be challenging.

In this book chapter, we draw attention on clinical manifestation and the most important laboratory investigations such us muscle histopathology, protein analysis, and genetic tests that can help in distinguishing between different forms of muscular dystrophy and could lead to an accurate diagnosis.

2. A general approach to the diagnosis of muscular dystrophy

The complexity and similarity of clinical manifestation of these conditions represent a challenge for getting an accurate diagnosis for patients. A complete diagnosis involved clinical examination and patient's medical history, blood tests (creatine kinase and serum transaminase levels), electromyography, muscle biopsy examination, and genetic tests [13–15].

Muscle biopsy had an important role in muscular dystrophy diagnosis and still provides essential information for diagnosis. Although in clinical observations, family history, muscle biopsy, and biochemical tests such as serum creatine kinase (CK) are still important tools for muscular dystrophy diagnosis, protein analysis and genetic study have an increasing importance in accurate establishing a diagnosis.

For several years, until the discovery of other muscle proteins, dystrophin was the only protein studied to establish a diagnosis of muscular dystrophy. It is also used today in the differential diagnosis between Duchenne muscular dystrophy (DMD) and Becker muscular dystrophy (BMD). In the last 10 years, genes involved in various types of autosomal recessive muscular dystrophy (LGMD) as well as in congenital muscle dystrophies have been identified [16–18].

Differentiation between recessive muscle dystrophies is much more difficult to achieve on the basis of clinical criteria because of phenotypic variability [19], different starting age of onset [20, 21], and a variable progression rate [22].

Identification of protein defect by immunohistochemistry and Western blotting allows firm and specific diagnosis in a wide variety of muscular dystrophies. However, while immunohistochemistry is very useful in identifying abnormal expression of primary protein deficiency, in genetically inherited recessive diseases, it is less useful for identifying primary defect in dominant diseases.

2.1 Clinical manifestations and symptoms for most common forms of muscular dystrophy

The patient's medical history and clinical examination allow the doctor to identify the signs and the specific symptoms of the diseases. A complete examination should include evaluation of movement and difficulty controlling movement, gait abnormalities, muscle strength, and the presence of weakness pattern, and also identification of the muscle groups affected.

While the most common sign for different types of muscular dystrophy is the progressive muscle weakness, the other features like age of disease onset, muscle group affected, and rate of progression are specific for each type of muscular dystrophy [21, 23].

2.1.1 Dystrophinopathies

Dystrophinopathies are recessive X-linked disorders caused by mutation in dystrophin gene [1]. Currently, they are recognized as a spectrum of disease with involvement of skeletal and cardiac muscle in different degree [24] and include Duchenne muscular dystrophy (DMD) and Becker muscular dystrophy (BMD), involving mostly skeletal muscles, and DMD-associated dilated cardiomyopathy (DCM), affecting preferentially the myocardium. The clinical picture in males with dystrophinopathies ranges from mild to severe. The mild forms consist of high level of CK in serum and muscle cramps with myoglobinuria. The severe forms include progressive muscle diseases (Duchenne muscle dystrophy, DMD, Becker muscle dystrophy, BMD).

2.1.1.1 Duchenne muscular dystrophy (DMD)

In DMD, affected boys are clinically normal at birth. The onset of clinical features is in early childhood with delayed motor milestones, including delayed independent walking, with a mean age of walking of 18 months, and difficulties in standing up from the floor. The most characteristic clinical features of DMD are general motor delays (42%) and gait problems including persistent toe walking and flat-footedness (30%) [25]. Patients with DMD have a waddling gait and difficulties in climbing stairs, running, jumping, and standing up due to proximal weakness [26]. They rise from a supine position using their arms (Gower maneuver). The boys have hypertrophic and firm calf muscles [27]. The disease is rapidly progressive, at the age of 12 years, most boys being wheelchair bound [25]. Subsequently, the function of upper extremity will be lost, and, by the age of 14–15 years, cardiomyopathy is a common feature [26]; during the teenage years, the patients will require assisted ventilation [27]. Progressive cardiomyopathy and respiratory complications represent the most common causes of death in patients with DMD. Typically, the death occurs by 30 years of age, but currently the life expectancy of these patients has been improved through an improved management of cardiorespiratory function [28].

Intellectual disability can be present in up to 27% of boys with DMD, and 44% of patients have learning disability [28]. Other psychiatric disorders reported in these patients include attention-deficit hyperactivity disorder (ADHD) (32%), anxiety (27%), and autism spectrum disorder (15%) [29].

2.1.1.2 Becker muscle dystrophy (BMD)

BMD is a milder form of muscular dystrophy characterized by skeletal muscle weakness with a later onset and a preservation of the gait for a longer period (age of 40–50 years) [25]. The patients present usually with high serum CK concentration, calf muscle hypertrophy, muscle cramps, myalgia, or with muscle weakness in the pelvic and shoulder girdles [26]. Cardiomyopathy is a common complication of BMD, the mean age of diagnosis being around 14, 6 years [28]. Heart failure represents the most common cause of death in BMD, at an age of mid-40s [23, 24].

2.1.2 Emery-Dreyfus muscular dystrophy (EDMD)

EDMD is a muscular disorder with different inheritance patterns: X-linked recessive or autosomal dominant or autosomal recessive [25, 26]. The clinical picture includes the classical triad: (i) early joint contractures, (ii) slowly progressive muscle weakness and wasting in humeroperoneal distribution (upper arm, lower legs), and (iii) cardiac disease (atrial-ventricular conduction anomalies, atrial arrhythmias) [27]. Usually, the clinical presentation is characterized by Achilles contractures with toe walking in childhood. Later, arm weakness and elbow contractures develop, associated with biceps or triceps wasting with sparing of deltoid muscle (a characteristic pattern called "Popeye arms." A rigid spine is also present causing a severe lumbar lordosis [27].

2.1.3 Limb-girdle muscular dystrophies (LGMDs)

LGMDs represent a group of muscular conditions with autosomal dominant or autosomal recessive inheritance, characterized by a typical pattern of slowly progressive, proximal weakness which involves shoulder and pelvic girdle muscles [18, 19]. Different subtypes of LGMDs have been described, with a wide clinical spectrum affecting various age groups. LGMDs with autosomal dominant inheritance are referred as LGMDs1 and recessive forms, as LGMDs2. LGMDs1 forms have, generally, a later onset and a milder course compared with autosomal recessive forms [29].

The most affected muscle groups are proximal muscles, namely, the muscles of the shoulders, upper arms, pelvis, and thighs. The clinical picture can vary among different subtypes of FSHD, even within the same family [29]. The onset of clinical features can be at any age and worsen with time. The first symptoms include abnormal gait (waddling gait, walking on the feet balls) and difficulties in running and standing up [29]. The muscle weakness slowly progresses, and, in later stage of the disease, the patients may be wheelchair bound. Other clinical features include scapular wings, lumbar lordosis, scoliosis, calf muscle hypertrophy and joint stiffness, that restrict movement of the elbows, hips, knees, and ankles [30]. Cardiomyopathy was reported in some forms of LGMD, and some patients may present respiratory difficulties which can vary from mild to severe. In some rare forms of LGMD, intellectual disability has been reported [31].

2.1.4 Facioscapulohumeral muscular dystrophy (FSHD)

FSHD is a genetic muscular disorder with autosomal dominant inheritance and a late onset; the disease has a slow progression and a high degree of phenotypic variability and side-to-side asymmetry [30]. The muscle weakness involves initial, facial, scapular, and proximal limb muscles (mimetic muscles, serratus anterior, rhomboid muscles, biceps, and triceps) [21]. The most frequent initial symptom is the inability to lift arms over shoulder height. Then, the weakness progress to lower limbs, typically the distal musculature first (tibialis anterior and gastrocnemius), and later more proximal muscles (quadriceps and hamstrings) and the pelvic girdle are involved [21]. The abdominal and paraspinal muscles can be affected, causing an exaggerated lumbar lordosis or camptocormia (bent spine syndrome) [22]. Pectus excavatum is another common feature in FSHD [22]. The risk to become wheelchair bound is high in the second decade for patients with a more severe infantile form and after the age of 50 years in about 20% of patients [23].

The respiratory involvement varies from 0 to 13% of patients with FSHD in different studies [24] and is caused by the loss of core/trunk muscles. It is present mostly in patients with pelvic girdle weakness who are wheelchair bound or with a marked paraspinal involvement or kyphoscoliosis. Between 1 and 8% of patients with FSHD require mechanical ventilation [23].

Cardiac involvement is not common in FSHD. 5–10% of patients can present supraventricular arrhythmias, mostly asymptomatic [25]; an incomplete right bundle branch block has been found in approximately one-third of patients in one study [26], with no significant progression.

Some extramuscular manifestations have been described in patients with FSHD, almost always in the cases with the smallest number of residual D4Z4 units. They include retinal vascular changes (peripheral telangiectasia); Coats disease, a severe retinal vasculopathy characterized by aneurysmal dilatations and exudation, which can cause retinal detachment or blindness; loss of high-frequency hearing, usually asymptomatic; hearing loss; and intellectual disability and seizures in infants with FSHD [32, 33].

A careful, complete, and thorough clinical examination along with laboratory investigations provides more information necessary for management of patients with muscular dystrophy, differentiates between the type of muscular dystrophy, and directs to subsequent analyses.

2.2 Laboratory investigations

When a muscular dystrophy is suspected, blood enzyme test and a variety of laboratory test can be used for confirmation of clinical diagnosis. The blood serum samples are used to determine the level of specific enzymes known to have a high blood serum levels when a dystrophic process is present:

i. Creatine kinase (CK) also known as creatine phosphokinase (CPK), an intracellular enzyme found with relative predominance in skeletal muscle, is considered as the most specific and sensitive marker of muscle disease. Normal reference value of CK ranges between 60 and 174 IU/L into blood serum [13, 14]. Elevated level of CK could suggest a muscle disease before symptoms of muscular dystrophy become evident [33, 34]. In early stages of the muscle disease, CK levels are 20–300 times greater than normal levels and tend to decrease with the muscle damage [15]. In male DMD patients, the serum CK level is markedly elevated due to muscle degeneration [17] with less elevation level noted in BMD patients. Recent studies show that losses of lung function in DMD patients determine the high level of CK in blood serum [35].

The level of CK has been found higher in other types of MD like limb-girdle muscular dystrophy (LGMD) [17] and could serve as useful indicator being able to discriminate between autosomal recessive and dominant types of LGMD, knowing that CK level recessive types of MD are higher than dominant ones. Also, evaluation of CK level is a useful screening tool for female DMD carrier.

It is interesting to note that not all cases of MD show a high level of CK. For example, in Ullrich congenital muscular dystrophy, Emery-Dreifuss muscular dystrophy, and Bethlem myopathy, the level of CK may be normal or slightly increased [22].

ii. Aldolase, transaminases (alanine aminotransferase ALT and aspartate aminotransferase AST), and lactate dehydrogenase (LDH) are other muscle enzymes also reported with a rise level in blood serum [18] when a muscular dystrophy is suspected.

Also, from the blood collected on anticoagulant (EDTA), total genomic DNA is isolated for further genetic tests used to confirm the diagnosis.

Other laboratory tests like electromyography, magnetic resonance imaging (MRI), combined with muscle biopsy, and genetic tests contribute for toward a diagnosis.

2.3 Muscle biopsy

The assessment of skeletal muscle biopsy is an essential procedure for an accurate diagnosis when a muscle disease is suspected, providing evidence of pathological changes in muscle and guides for appropriate tests.

2.3.1 Muscle histopathological analysis

Even though the muscle biopsy is a highly invasive procedure, the data gained from it has the utmost importance for histopathological diagnosis and is an essential component in the diagnosis of muscle disorders that could identify the cause of the disease process and distinguish between different types of muscular dystrophy. The overall structure of the tissue as well as all specific histological features of dystrophic muscle can be observed by hematoxylin and eosin (H&E) staining performed on frozen sections sampled from the quadriceps or deltoid muscle. Generally, the features observed in all dystrophic muscle biopsy include fibers' size variation, round shape muscle fibers, the presence of atrophy, regenerating and degenerating fibers, splitting of fibers, proliferation of the connective tissue, and increased number of internal nuclei. In the end phases of the disease, the fibers are replaced by adipose tissue [36]. Histopathological changes differ widely in severity among the types of muscular dystrophy, as well as among allelic variants of the same genotype. Also, some features are specific for each type of muscular dystrophy. For example, lobulated fibers are characteristic for LGMD 2A; a high variability in fibers'size is specific for LGMD 1C, and increased internally nuclei are specific for myotonic dystrophy; the presence of rimmed vacuoles suggests a myotilinopathy, while prominent vacuoles are found in LGMD [36]. With all signs, none of the specific forms of muscular dystrophy can be diagnosed just based only on histological analysis.

Also, the muscle biopsy analysis can not only denote the specific genetic cause of the disease but can also provide clues for further investigation. In combination with protein analysis, the genetic investigations can provide an accurate diagnosis.

2.3.2 Protein analysis

The study of muscle protein expression is important for diagnosis, for genotype-phenotype correlations, and to identify possible genetic defect [37–39]. There are many methods used for the study of muscle protein expression [40], but the most used are immunostaining methods (immunohistochemistry or similar methods immunofluorescence and immunoblotting/Western blotting (WB)). Both methods use labeled antibodies for a specific muscle protein involved in a type of muscular dystrophy. While the immunohistochemistry/immunofluorescence method is used to identify the localization and relative abundance of the proteins, in tissue cryosections, the WB method is useful to detect the total amount of proteins as well as the normal or reduced size of the proteins in homogenized sample.

2.3.2.1 Immunofluorescence (IF)

In the past, the diagnosis of muscular dystrophy consisted only on clinical assessment, serum *CK levels*, and histological investigations of muscle biopsy [41, 42].

The discovery in 1986 of the first muscle protein involved in a type of muscular dystrophy, dystrophin [43], has later led to the identification of the dystrophin-associated protein complex (DAPC) [44] and other additional proteins from the muscle cytosol (calpain 3, TRIM32) [45], from extracellular matrix (a2-laminin, collagen VI) from the sarcomere (telethonin, myotilin, titin, nebulin) [46]. Each of these proteins is involved in a type of muscular dystrophy; so far over 40 types of muscular dystrophy are known [47].

The development of specific antibodies (Abs) for affected proteins has improved the diagnosis for these diseases, over time. Now, there are many immunohistochemical protocols based on the use of specific antibodies for antigen localization through antigen-antibody interaction.

IF or fluorescent antibody staining is a helpful routinely technique widely used to determine the localization of fluorescent-tagged protein and changes in protein expression on a cryosection (presence, reduced, and absence). It is also used to investigate muscle architecture.

A large array of antibodies directed against different muscle protein is now available for current diagnosis and allows the use of these techniques for the diagnosis of many muscle disorders (see **Table 1**).

The use of antibodies directed against muscle protein *is useful to gain information about integrity of muscle complexes, secondary reduction of proteins, and also gene function by compared normal and affected patients* (see **Figure 1**) [48].

In addition, IF method identifies also the secondary reduction and overexpression of closely protein levels [49]. For example, utrophin, an autosomal protein which presents around 80% sequence homology to dystrophin [50, 51] and localized in normal skeletal muscle at the neuromuscular junction (NMJ) [52], is overexpressed in dystrophinopathies (see **Figure 2**) [53, 54]. Mutations in one sarcoglycan often lead to reduced expression of other sarcoglycans [49], and reductions of dysferlin (see **Figure 3**) are observed in other forms of muscular dystrophy such as calpainopathy, caveolinopathy, and anoctaminopathy [55].

However, IF is not always helpful in diagnosis of all forms of MD. For example, in LGMD 2A some available antibodies have no immunoreactions on the sections. Few studies tried to analyze calpain 3 on cryosections but, because of rapid degradation of calpain 3 after harvesting, concluded that immunostaining analysis alone does not predict the presence of CAPN3 mutations [40]. However, the staining of other proteins such us dystrophin and sarcoglycans which appear normal on cryosections by IF could be informative for further analysis.

Also, in dominant forms LGMD1B caused by changes in the *LMNA* gene which encode for lamin A/C, immunostaining of cryosection reveals normal expression even in the presence of a mutation [56].

Antibody	Manufacturer	Clone	Dilution for cryosection	Dilution for Western blot
Dystrophin C-terminus	Novocstra	Dy8/6C5	1:40	1:200
Dystrophin N-terminus	Novocstra	Dy10/12B2	1:50	1:50
Dystrophin rod domain	Novocstra	Dy4/6D3	1:20	1:200
Utrophin	Novocstra	DRP3/20C	1:50	1:200
Calpain 3	Novocstra	2C4	—	1:100
Calpain 3	Novocstra	12A2	—	1:50
Caveolin 3	Santa Cruz	A-3	1:50	1:200
Dysferlin	Novocstra	Ham1/7B6	1:50	1:100
α-Sarcoglycan	Novocstra	Ad1/20A6	1:50	1:100
β-Sarcoglycan	Novocstra	BSarc/5B1	1:50	1:100
γ-Sarcoglycan	Novocstra	35DAG/21B5	1:50	1:100
Merosin	Novocstra	Mer3/22B2	1:50	1:50

Table 1.
Details of the most used antibodies in muscular dystrophy diagnosis.

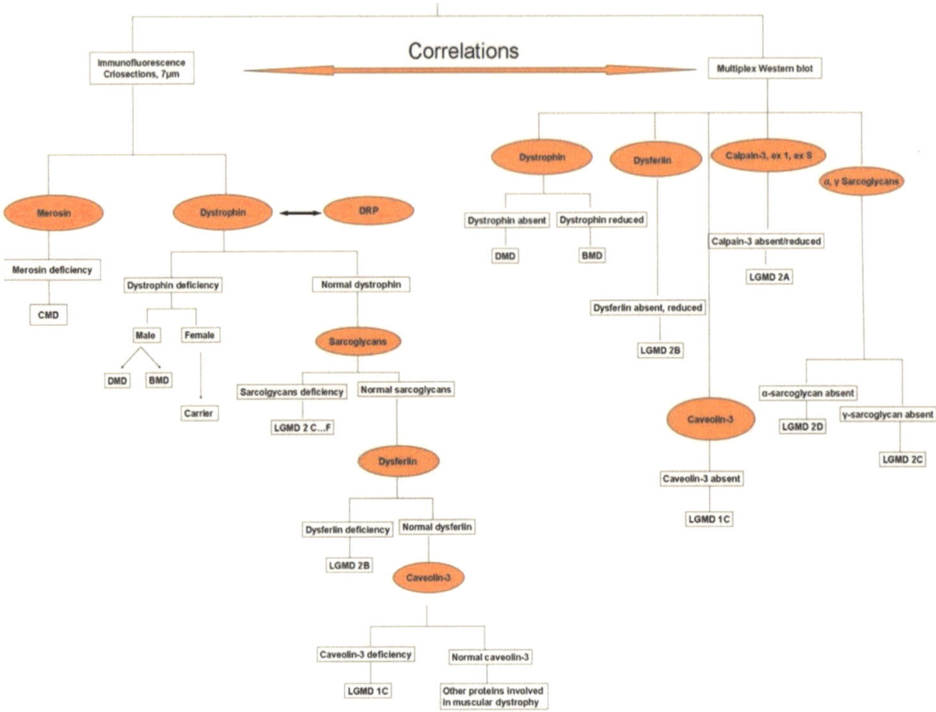

Figure 1.
Workflow chart for muscle protein analysis in muscular dystrophy diagnostic process.

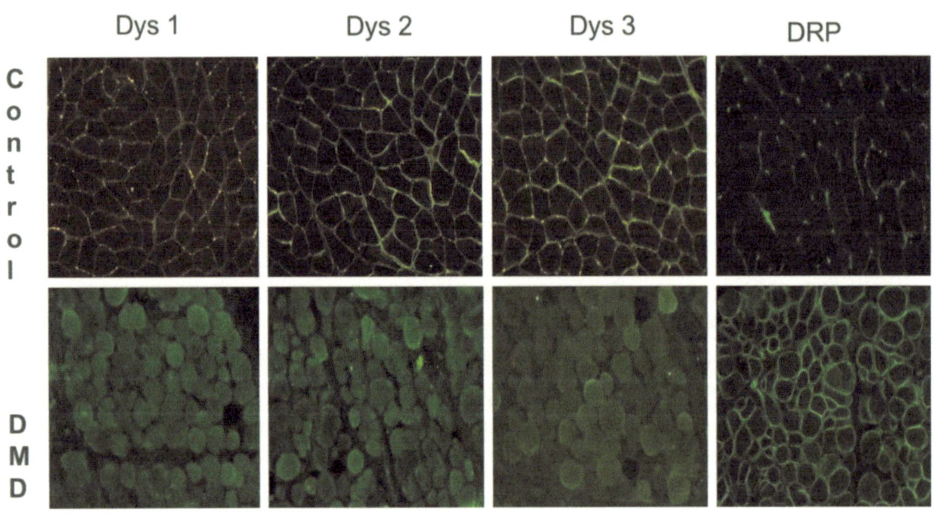

Figure 2.
Representative immunofluorescent staining from dystrophin and utrophin in normal human (control) and DMD and BMD skeletal muscle.

It is important to note that to obtain good results in protein evaluation by IF is a necessary investigation of the integrity of muscle fiber membrane by analysis of spectrin [54, 57].

All these facts suggest the difficulty of identification with accuracy of a type of MD based only on histochemical findings and immunofluorescence analysis and indicate a further investigation of proteins using immunoblot analysis.

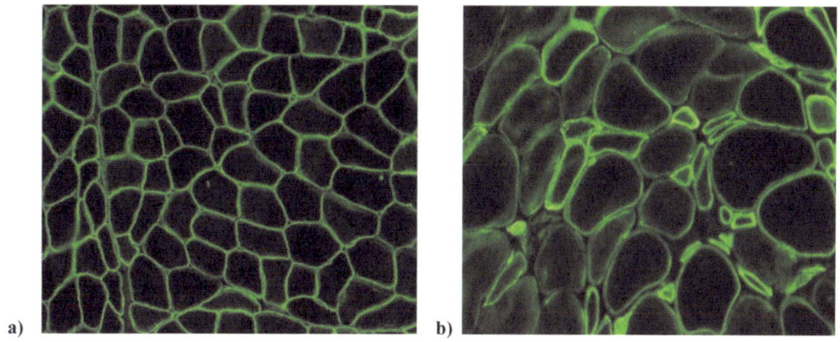

Figure 3.
Immunofluorescent staining of dysferlin in normal control muscle and patient with LGMD 2B: (a) expression of dysferlin from normal patients; (b) reduced expression of dysferlin around some muscle fiber; the presence of regenerating fiber.

2.3.2.2 Multiplex Western blotting

Western blot (WB), also called immunoblot, is a semiquantitative method used to detect specific proteins from cell lysate samples or tissue homogenates using specific antibodies [58].

Due to higher sensitivity and specificity of the method, WB brings more information about proteins that cannot be offered by other immunoassay techniques. The WB technique is an extremely powerful technique which gives information about the presence, absence, and size of the proteins, identifying the proteins with abnormal molecular weight [59, 60].

Usually, this analytical method involved three major processes [61]: (i) separation of proteins into a SDS-polyacrylamide gel based on their molecular weight; (ii) protein blotting on a nitrocellulose or polyvinylidene fluoride (PVDF) membrane; and (iii) visualization of the protein of interest by incubation of membrane with specific primary antibody and then labeled by secondary antibody conjugate with an enzyme.

For the preparation of tissue lysates, around 20–80 mg of muscle tissue are required which may be a significant part of a severely affected muscle. Cooper et al. [62] reported in 2003 obtaining of the lysate from 16 mg muscle tissue using a single cryosection (8 μm thick, 10 mm^2).

Given the complexity of muscular dystrophies, in recent years, has become a necessity in the analysis and comparison of the expression of multiple target proteins involved in a specific pathology.

Also, the technology has improved over time going from the detection of a single protein to identification of multiple proteins in complex samples using a biphasic polyacrylamide gel systems and a cocktail of primary antibodies [63]. In our laboratory, polyacrylamide gel system is performed as previously described [63] with some modifications [64, 65] which permitted separation of the large proteins more than 200 kDa (e.g., dystrophin) in the top part of the gel while and smaller proteins under 150 kDa (e.g., calpain 3), in the bottom. The intensity and thickness of the specific protein bands correspond to the relative abundance of protein of interest. The amount of target protein is determined by comparing stained band of control with the patients. Quantification of protein based on densitometry of bands using ImageJ software provides information about the relative level of protein in muscle.

In DMD patients, the total absence of the bands for dystrophin at 427 kDa is observed, while BMD patients show a reduced intensity of the bands for dystrophin (see **Figure 4**).

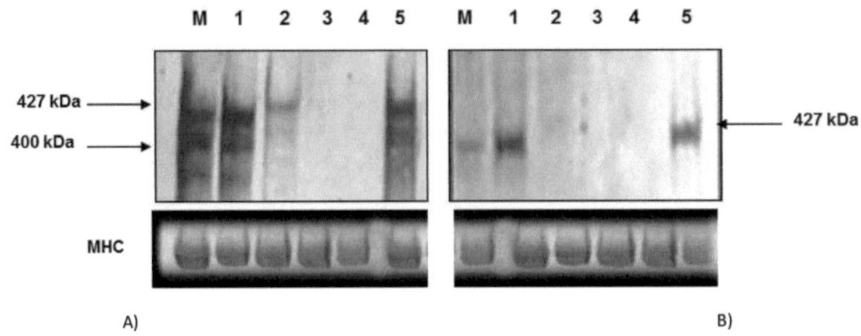

Figure 4.
Representative Western blotting analysis of muscle homogenates from four patients with muscular dystrophy: (A) nitrocellulose membrane labeled with antibody against rod domain of dystrophin (NCL-Dys1). (B) Blot labeled with antibody against C-terminus domain of dystrophin (NCL-Dys2); M-normal control; lane 1-MD with normal expression of dystrophin; lane 2-BMD; lane 3-DMD, absence of dystrophin band; lane 4-DMD; lane 5 MD with normal expression of dystrophin. MHC—Corresponding myosin heavy chain bands on the post-blotted gel, stained with Coomassie blue.

WB plays an important role in distinguishing between DMD and BMD patients especially for patients with discordant phenotype (do no respect reading frame rule).

Analysis by WB of calpain 3, protein found to be involved in LGMD 2A, could show a total or a reduced intensity of bands at 94 kDa. There are cases with LGMD 2A which displayed normal or almost normal bands for calpain 3 compared with control (see **Figure 5**).

This fact suggests a poor specificity of WB analysis for this protein [66]. Also, false-negative results provided by WB can be found in analysis of dysferlin when this protein is accumulated in the cytoplasm, and deficiency of lamin A/C could not be identified in all patients with LMNA mutations [67].

However, for these proteins, genetic analyses are required to confirm the exact diagnosis.

Western blot has the advantage of simultaneous analysis of several proteins which reduced cost and time for analysis. This method is useful in differential diagnosis of muscular dystrophies providing information on the relative location of mutation.

2.4 DNA diagnosis methods

The identification and characterization of genetic defect involved in pathology is often essential both for diagnosis and treatment options as well as in predicting

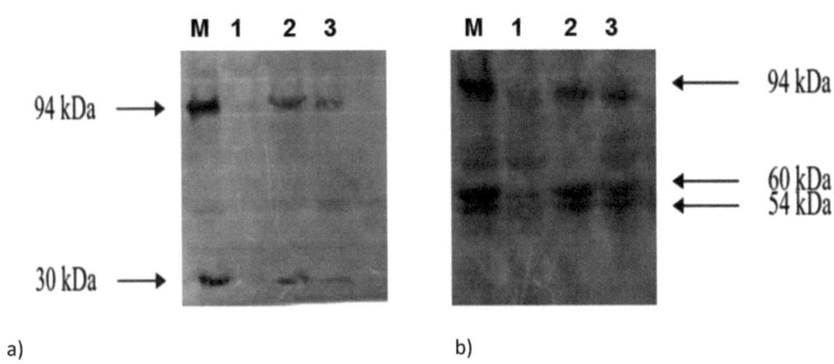

Figure 5.
Calpain 3 band patterns on WB. Representative Western blotting analysis of muscle homogenates from three patients analyzed with antibody against calpain 3. (a) Nitrocellulose membrane labeled with antibody against calpain 3 NCL-CALP-2C4 detects bands at 90 and 30 kDa in normal patients. (b) Nitrocellulose membrane labeled with antibody against calpain 3 NCL-CALP-12A2 detects bands at 90 kDa and two bands at 60 and 30 kDa in normal patients.

disease prognosis. Additionally, diagnostic accuracy leads to more specific genetic counseling for families and possible preimplantation prenatal diagnosis.

The great technological advances in molecular assays over the last 20 years have led to the identification of the molecular genetic cause for many forms of muscular dystrophy. This advance enabled, thus, the diagnosis of muscular dystrophy to evolve from the analysis of 20 exons out of 79 exons within hotspot region of *DMD* gene by PCR Multiplex [68–70] to multiple gene analysis using next-generation sequencing (NGS) technique.

Different forms of muscular dystrophy are caused by a variety of mutations that occurred in many human genes. Mutations that occurred in gene that encode for proteins from DAPC are responsible for many types of muscular dystrophy. The most common types of mutations involve large rearrangement (deletion and duplication) and point mutations. A correct characterization gene mutation for each type of muscular dystrophy represents the key for genotype-phenotype correlation.

Here, we describe some of the more used molecular techniques in the muscular dystrophy diagnosis.

2.4.1 Multiplex ligation-dependent probe amplification (MLPA)

Among the different methods used for detection of gene deletions and duplication, the MLPA assay is the most used due to rapid analysis up to 45 different DNA fragments in a single PCR amplification with only a single primer pair [71] and low amounts of genomic DNA. In addition to large deletions and duplications, MLPA may also identify single exon deletion. This apparent result should be always checked by an alternative method avoiding false-positive results that can occur in the presence of a single-nucleotide variation in a gene. This method proves its usefulness for female's carrier screening as well as for prenatal testing [72].

Because require equipments that exist in most molecular diagnosis laboratory (a thermocycler and a capillary electrophoresis), is a very cost-effective method widely used for both diagnostic and research.

Data analysis can be done by using the free MLPA data analysis software Coffalyser (MRC-Holland, Amsterdam, the Netherlands) or additional software such as MLPAinter [73] or GeneMapper v4.0 software [74].

The advantages of MLPA method for diagnosis are (i) low input of DNA required; (ii) the high specificity and sensitivity, the method being able to distinguish sequences differing in only one nucleotide; and (iii) plenty of MLPA kits available for different genes involved in muscle pathology such as CAPN3, DYSF, SGCA, SGCB, SGCD, SGCG, and FKRP.

2.4.2 High-resolution melting curve analysis (hrMCA)

High-resolution melting curve analysis (hrMCA) is a highly sensitive molecular post PCR method introduced in 1997 by Wittwer et al. [75, 76], to identify pathogenic variants in nucleic acid sequences. The improvement of real-time equipment regarding highly controlled temperature transitions, data acquisition software to monitor and analyze the melting, as well as the development of a new functional class of dyes have made this technology possible.

HRM analysis starts with PCR amplification of the region of interest with specific primers in the presence of a specialized double-stranded DNA (dsDNA) fluorescent binding dye.

The method is based on the DNA property of dissociating (or melting) from double-stranded DNA into single-stranded DNA (ssDNA) when exposed to a gradual temperature [77, 78]. The melting process can be real time monitored by measuring the gradually diminishing amount of fluorescence during DNA strand dissociation. The presence of a mutation in PCR products determines a modification in the shape of DNA melting curves comparative with melting profile of the wild type (normal) DNA (see **Figure 6**).

HR-MCA is a rapid and accurate method for detection of genetic variation in population. Although HR-MCA is not locus specific, it can become a tool of choice for point mutations screening after identification of large mutation (deletion and duplications) by MLPA. The sequencing of the fragments with abnormal melting profile only, identified by HR-MCA, *reduces costs* and waiting *time* per archived results.

2.4.3 Sanger sequencing

All point mutations identified by HR-MCA method need to be confirmed by sequencing. Sequencing, the most widely used approach for DNA analysis, remains the "gold standard" for mutation analysis.

The Sanger DNA sequencing method is applied to *determine the* sequence of a DNA molecule and to identify the subtle mutations in samples compared with a reference sequence [79, 80].

Because a lot of muscle proteins associated with different forms of muscular dystrophy are extremely large, full gene analysis using Sanger sequencing can lead to higher costs and is time-consuming for analysis. The method finds its usefulness in the analysis of small gene composed of only few exons in which the frequency of point mutation is higher. For instance gene that encode for sarcoglycans (e.g., *SGCA* 10 exons, *SGCB* 6 exons, *SGCG* 10 exons), for calpain 3 *(CAPN3* 26 exons),

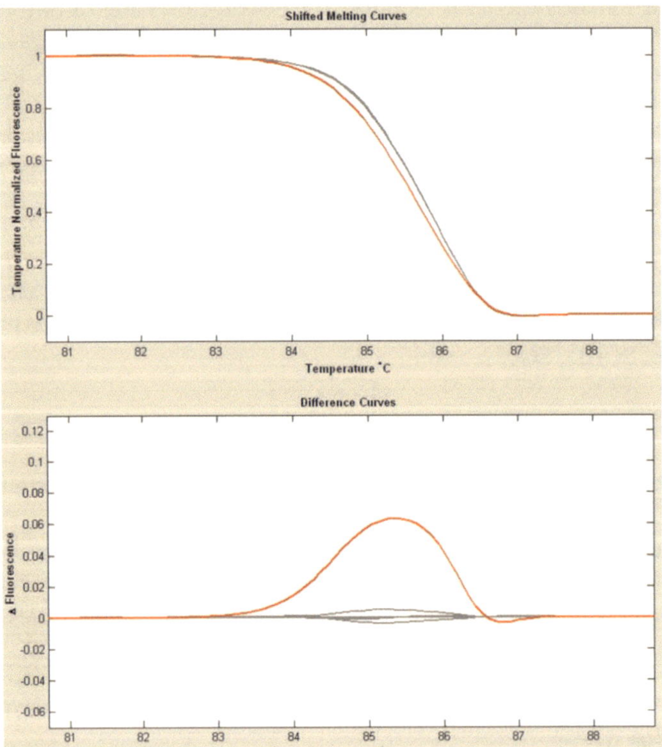

Figure 6.
Representative high-resolution melting curve analysis which reveals difference in melting shape between wild type and variant sequence.

and for dysferlin (*DYSF* 58 exons) [81] that are associated with LGMDs, is more suitable for sequencing.

Due to overlapping clinical symptoms and many possible genetic causes for LGMDs, obtaining a *diagnosis is* often *difficult*. Next-generation sequencing becomes a valuable option for an accurate diagnosis due to ability to analyze a large number of targets.

In *DMD* gene (79 exons), a high frequency of point mutations around 35% was reported [82]. Screening of this huge gene for point mutation is difficult to perform; therefore it is necessary to select only genomic regions that contain the variants [83].

However, the combined technology MLPA for identification of large deletions and duplication followed by HR-MCA and sequencing is a robust algorithm for diagnosis for male muscular dystrophy patients as well as for female carrier and also for prenatal diagnosis.

2.5 Diagnosis algorithm in the most common forms of MD

2.5.1 Dystrophinopathies

The presence of clinical symptoms in a male child presented in Cap 2.1 along with *increased* serum *levels of CK*, *transaminase* enzymes or aldolase should trigger the diagnostic investigation for dystrophinopathies [11]. When DMD or BMD is suspected, diagnostic recommendation as first investigation is the screening of *DMD* gene for deletions and duplications by MLPA. The presence of a mutation in gene confirms the dystrophinopathies diagnosis.

A large number of research studies highlight the utility of MLPA as detection methods for *DMD* gene [84–86] which is the largest gene (2.2 Mb) of the human genome.

Many different types of mutations that occurred in the *DMD* gene, encoding for the cytoskeletal protein, dystrophin, are responsible for both severe disease Duchenne muscular dystrophy (DMD) and the milder form of the disease Becker muscular dystrophy (BMD). The difference in disease severity between the two phenotypes, DMD and BMD, can be explained by the "reading frame rule" proposed by Monaco in 1988 [87]. According to this theory, DMD is caused by mutations which disrupt the reading frame, and no protein will be synthesized, while for BMD phenotype the mutations do not affect the reading frame leading to the synthesis of a smaller and semi-functional dystrophin protein.

Previously reported studies have shown that all over the world, deletions of one or more exons are most common mutation in dystrophinopathies (60–65%), followed by duplications (5–8%) and point mutations (30–35%) [88]. Around 90% from all dystrophinopathies cases present worldwide respect reading frame rule. For the remaining 10% as well as for patients with discordant phenotype, additional analyses are required for an accurate diagnosis.

Because the mutations have been observed across all exons of the gene with a higher incidence of mutation in two "hotspots" regions between exons 2–20 and 45–50 [85, 89], MLPA method proves its utility for the molecular diagnosis of dystrophinopathies, by simultaneous screening of all 79 exons of DMD gene for large intragenic rearrangements [90]. All deletion and duplications identified should be checked *for* the validity of the *reading frame rule on* http://www.dmd.nl.

If no deletions and duplication are identified, the *DMD* gene should be investigated for point mutations [91] by hrMCA followed by sequencing of exons with a modification of melting curve only. Full characterization of the mutation (type, size, and position) is important in identification of patients that are eligible for specific mutation gene therapy [89].

If a muscle biopsy is the tool of choice as first step in analysis routine, histochemical staining and dystrophin analysis by immunohistochemistry/immunofluorescence and Western blot confirm or not the dystrophinopathies diagnosis based on the difference in the expression of dystrophin.

Analysis by IF of dystrophin in muscle samples using three monoclonal mouse antibodies against three domains of protein (C-terminal, rod domain, and N-terminal) revealed the localization of protein at the sarcolemmal level of skeletal muscle fibers and displays a normal expression of intensity signal around each muscle fiber. In DMD patients, dystrophin is absent or severely reduced, while BMD patients displayed a variable expression of signal for dystrophin. Also, labeling of dystrophin on sections plays a critical role in identification process of the DMD female carriers which display a mosaic pattern of dystrophin expression.

Western blot as additional method confirms the diagnostic.

It's important to note that the protein result should be confirmed by genetic analysis.

2.5.2 Limb-girdle muscular dystrophies

Limb-girdle muscular dystrophies (LGMD) are a highly clinically and genetically heterogeneous group of muscle disorders that affect in both males' and females' voluntary muscles of the pelvic and shoulder areas [92].

Major advances in last decades, both in neuromuscular disorders field and diagnostic assays, made that many genes associated with LGMDs to be found such us: CAPN3 (encode for calpain 3), DYSF (encode for dysferlin), FKRP (encode for fukutin), SGCA, SGCB, SGCG, and SGCD (that encode for the α-, β-, γ-, and δ-sarcoglycan), and more than 30 forms of LGMDs to be characterized [11, 37]. However, a significant number of patients clinically diagnosed with LGMDs remain molecularly uncharacterized [93].

Based on their inheritance pattern were classified in dominant (type 1 LGMD) and recessive forms (type 2 LGMD) [94].

Giving the complexity of the clinical symptoms and different genes involved, a diagnosis algorithm for these pathologies is still waiting, but comprehensive guidelines for identifying these disorders have been published. The initial evaluation of a patient involves clinical examination, followed by laboratory test such as serum creatine kinase measurements, genetic tests, and muscle biopsy analysis. CK level can vary from lower level in dominantly inherited LGMD forms to very high level in recessively inherited forms [95].

All these diagnostic approaches should be sufficient to accurately predict the correct form of LGMDs. In the last years, the increasing use of next-generation sequencing technology for simultaneous analysis of known LGMD-related genes improved diagnostic rate and offered opportunity to identified new disease-related genes [96]. However, this technology is extremely expensive and is not yet available in all the molecular diagnostic laboratories.

If the clinical features, laboratory tests, and other investigations such as electromyography, magnetic resonance, or ultrasound imaging suggest a LGMD, muscle biopsy [97] may be considered an appropriate test to start the investigation.

Routine histochemical stains will display variable degree of typically dystrophic feature characteristic for LGMD: variation in fiber size, degeneration and regeneration fiber, *presence of internal nuclei*, and *increased* endomysial *fibrosis* [37, 40].

Disease prediction based on clinical and histochemical *tests alone* is difficult to achieve, so immunohistochemical stains (IHC or IF) of specific muscle proteins involved in LGMDs (calpain 3, dysferlin, caveolin3, the sarcoglycans, myotilin, lamin A/C, etc.) provides useful information about the presence, absence and changes in protein expression. Muscle biopsy is not always informative taken into account the secondary protein reduction in addition to the primary protein deficiency but can guide to targeted genetic tests. Although genetic testing can be expensive, it will identify the exact defect of the disease. Being composed only few exons and considering that LGMDs could have many possible genetic causes, the sequencing of genes is the most suitable method of choices for diagnosis.

Autosomal dominant LGMDs' form is quiet rare in population. Recessive forms are more common and studied. The most commonly recessive form of LGMDs and the most studied are LGMD 2A (calpainopathy) and LGMD 2B (dysferlinopathy).

2.5.2.1 Limb-girdle muscular dystrophy 2A (LGMD2A)

LGMD 2A is the most common form of limb-girdle muscular dystrophy accounting for about 30% of all LGMDs, caused by mutation in CAPN3 gene which encodes for calcium sensitive dependent protease-calpain 3 protein.

Besides the clinical manifestation and laboratory investigation of serum enzymes presented above, for characterization of this condition, searching for mutations in CAPN3 gene in correlation with protein calpain 3 investigations by Western blot represents the "gold standard" in LGMD2A. The identification of the mutations in CAPN3 gene is most often difficult due to many genetic variations which appear in this gene and the position they have in the gene.

The improvement of next-generation sequencing technology (NGS), which screens genomic DNA for a large number of genes involved in neuromuscular disease, makes LGMD diagnosis easier to achieve. However, in most laboratories, the diagnosis starts with screening for mutation by direct Sanger sequencing analysis of the 24 exons of the CAPN3 gene. With this method more than 95% cases are diagnosed. Even if this analysis is successful, in most cases, there are not always identify large deletions and duplications as well as intronic splice mutations [98]. This fact shows importance of screening for large genomic rearrangements by MLPA, the most cost-effective techniques. Sanger sequencing combined with MLPA leads to an increase in the mutation detection rate and remains one of the most valuable diagnostic tools. Therefore, when DNA analysis is not conclusive, a muscle biopsy is required for protein analyses.

Until this moment, only few studies reported the success of immunohistochemical technique application for the diagnosis of LGMD using calp3d/12A2 and calp2C4 antibodies [40, 99] and demonstrated the localization of calpain 3 in myofibrils and myonuclei.

Nowadays, it is widely accepted that WB, even if it does not have a high accuracy, is the most suitable method for calpain 3 analysis.

In general, for analysis, two antibodies which produce characteristic patterns of bands are used: NCL-CALP-2C4 directed against exon 1 which recognizes the full-sized protein at 94 kDa and additional band at 30 kDa and NCL-CALP-12A2 against exon 8 that recognizes also to the full-sized protein at 94 kDa and additionally bands doublet at 60 and 54 kDa. An example of normal calpain on blot is shown in **Figure** 5.

Identification and interpretation of the pattern of bands obtained on WB by using the two antibodies for calpain 3 provide useful information about protein expression in muscle. Generally, it is widely accepted that the complete absence of all specific calpain 3 bands on blot is specific for LGMD2A diagnosis and is due to a primary defect in CAPN3 [100]. The presence of a normal amount of calpain-3 protein on blot does not exclude the LGMD 2A diagnosis. The normal amount of calpain-3 protein on blot in patients with LGMD 2A was reported [101] by several studies. The possible explanation of normal expression but functionally inactive protein is due to a functional enzyme defect that impairs the autolytic or proteolytic activity of protein without elimination of protein from the muscle [102, 103].

The reduction is more difficult to interpret because calpain-3 appears to reduce in amount as secondary effect in other forms of muscular dystrophies such as dysferlinopathies [40] and titinopathies [81, 92].

Even if muscle calpain-3 results on blot should always be confirmed by mutation analysis, Western blot remains one of the most valuable diagnostic tools in LGMDs allowing for the simultaneous analysis of multiple proteins, identifying both the primary defect and the secondary reductions.

3. Summary and future directions

For most forms of muscular dystrophy, the diagnosis is still challenging, and a multidisciplinary approach is always required. Only a good knowledge of protein and gene involved in pathology can provide the correct diagnosis and is essential for therapeutic interventions. New genetic therapies under development like exon skipping which tried to restore the reading frame with antisense oligonucleotides and to transform severe DMD phenotype in a less severe phenotype require a good characterization of the mutation.

When clinical symptoms are combined with protein analysis by immunofluorescence and Western blot, and with high-throughput DNA molecular technique such us MLPA, hrMCA, and sequencing, the diagnostic capabilities greatly improve and can provide an accurate diagnosis.

A defined genetic diagnosis is important for an appropriate treatment and genetic counseling as well as inclusion of patients in further clinical trials.

Acknowledgements

This study is funded by the Ministry of Research and Innovation in Romania, under Program 1, The Improvement of the National System of Research and Development, Subprogram 1.2—Institutional Excellence—Projects of Excellence Funding in RDI, Contract No. 7PFE/16.10.2018, and National Program 31N/2016/ PN16.22.02.05.

Conflict of interest

The authors declare that they have no competing interests.

Acronyms and abbreviations

BMD	Becker muscular dystrophy
CK	creatine kinase
CMD	congenital muscular dystrophy
DAPC	dystrophin-associated protein complex
DMD	Duchenne muscular dystrophy
DM	myotonic dystrophy (DM1 Type 1, DM2 Type 2)
EDMD	emery-Dreyfus muscular dystrophy
FCMD	fukuyama congenital muscular dystrophy
FSHD	facioscapulohumeral muscular dystrophy

DOI: http://dx.doi.org/10.5772/intechopen.85339

hrMCA	high-resolution melting curve analysis
IF	immunofluorescence
IHC	immunohistochemistry
LGMD	limb-girdle muscular dystrophy
MD	muscular dystrophy
MEB	muscle-eye-brain disease
MLPA	multiplex ligation-dependent probe amplification
WB	Western blot

Author details

Gisela Gaina[1,2]*, Magdalena Budisteanu[1], Emilia Manole[1] and Elena Ionica[2]

1 Victor Babes National Institute of Pathology, Bucharest, Romania

2 Department of Biochemistry and Molecular Biology, University of Bucharest, Bucharest, Romania

*Address all correspondence to: giselagaina@yahoo.com; giss_g@yahoo.com

References

[1] Emery AE. Population frequencies of inherited neuromuscular diseases—A world survey. Neuromuscular Disorders. 1991;**1**:19-29. DOI: 10.1016/0960-8966(91)90039-U

[2] Bushby K, Finkel R, et al. Diagnosis and management of Duchenne muscular dystrophy, part 1: Diagnosis, and pharmacological and psychosocial management. Lancet Neurology. 2010; **9**(1):77-93. DOI: 10.1016/S1474-4422(09)70271-6

[3] Nicholson LV, Johnson MA, Bushby KM, Gardner-Medwin D, Curtis A, Ginjaar IB. Integrated study of 100 patients with Xp21 linked muscular dystrophy using clinical, genetic, immunochemical, and histopathological data. Part 1. Trends across the clinical groups. Journal of Medical Genetics. 1993;**30**:728-736

[4] Brockington M, Blake DJ, et al. Mutations in the fukutin-related protein gene (FKRP) cause a form of congenital muscular dystrophy with secondary laminin alpha2 deficiency and abnormal glycosylation of alpha-dystroglycan. American Journal of Human Genetics. 2001;**69**(6):1198-1209. DOI: 10.1086/324412

[5] Brockington M, Sewry CA, et al. Assignment of a form of congenital muscular dystrophy with secondary merosin deficiency to chromosome 1q42. American Journal of Human Genetics. 2000;**66**(2):428-435. DOI: 10.1086/302775

[6] Angelini C, Fanin M, Freda MP, et al. The clinical spectrum of sarcoglycanopathies. Neurology. 1999; **52**:176-179

[7] Richard I, Broux O, Allamand V, et al. Mutations in the proteolytic enzyme calpain 3 cause limb-girdle muscular dystrophy typ. 2A. Cell. 1995;**81**:27-40

[8] Nardes F, Araújo AP, Ribeiro MG. Mental retardation in Duchenne muscular dystrophy. Jornal de Pediatria. 2012;**88**(1):6-16

[9] Mochizuki H, Miyatake S, Suzuki M, Shigeyama T, Yatabe K, Ogata K, et al. Mental retardation and lifetime events of Duchenne muscular dystrophy in Japan. Internal Medicine. 2008;**47**:1207-1210

[10] Ensenauer RE, Michels VV, et al. Genetic testing: Practical, ethical, and counseling considerations. Mayo Clinic Proceedings. 2005;**80**(1):63-73

[11] Bach JR. Management of Patients with Neuromuscular Disease. Philadelphia: Hanley & Belfus; 2004

[12] Gomez-Merino E, Bach JR. Duchenne muscular dystrophy: Prolongation of life by noninvasive ventilation and mechanically assisted coughing. American Journal of Physical Medicine & Rehabilitation. 2002;**81**: 411-415

[13] Fardeau M, Desguerre I. Diagnostic workup for neuromuscular diseases. Handbook of Clinical Neurology. 2013; **113**:1291-1297

[14] Rosalki SB. Serum enzymes in disease of skeletal muscle. Clinics in Laboratory Medicine. 1989;**9**:767-781

[15] Carbone I, Bruno C, Sotgia F, et al. Mutation in the CAV3 gene causes partial caveolin-3 deficiency and hyperCKemia. Neurology. 2000;**54**: 1373-1376

[16] Bushby K, Norwood F, Straub V. The limb-girdle muscular dystrophies—Diagnostic strategies. Biochimica et Biophysica Acta. 2007;**1772**(2):238-242

[17] Zhu Y, Zhang H, Sun H, Li Y, Deng L, Wen X, et al. Serum enzyme

profiles differentiate five types of muscular dystrophy. Disease Markers. 2015;**2015**:543282

[18] Sveen ML, Schwartz M, Vissing J. High prevalence and phenotype-genotype correlations of limb girdle muscular dystrophy typ. 2I in Denmark. Annals of Neurology. 2006;**59**:808-815

[19] Ginjaar IB, Kneppers AL, et al. Dystrophin nonsense mutation induces different levels of exon 29 skipping and leads to variable phenotypes within one BMD family. European Journal of Human Genetics. 2000;**8**(10):793-796

[20] Ciafaloni E, Kumar A, Liu K, Westfield C, Fox DJ, Caspers Conway KM, et al. Age at onset of first signs or symptoms predicts age at loss of ambulation in Duchenne and Becker muscular dystrophy: Data from the MD STARnet. Journal of Pediatric Rehabilitation Medicine. 2016;**9**(1):5-11

[21] Anthony A, Griggs RC. Overview of the muscular dystrophies. In: Handbook of Clinical Neurology (3rd Series). Vol. 101. Amsterdam, The Netherlands: Elsevier; 2011

[22] Romitti PA, Zhu Y, Puzhankara S, James KA, Nabukera SK, Zamba GK, et al. Prevalence of Duchenne and Becker muscular dystrophies in the United States. Pediatrics. 2015;**135**(3): 513-521

[23] Muntoni F, Torelli S, Ferlini A. Dystrophin and mutations: One gene, several proteins, multiple phenotypes. Lancet Neurology. 2003;**2**:731-740

[24] Zalaudek I, Bonelli RM, Koltringer P, Reisecker F, Wagner K. Early diagnosis in Duchenne muscular dystrophy. Lancet. 1999;**353**:1975

[25] Liang WC, Wang CH, Chou PC, Chen WZ, Jong YJ. The natural history of the patients with Duchenne muscular dystrophy in Taiwan: A medical center experience. Pediatrics and Neonatology. 2018;**59**:176-183

[26] Darras BT, Menache-Starobinski CC, Hinton V, Kunkel LM. Dystrophinopathies. In: Darras BT, Jones HR, Ryan MM, De Vivo DC, editors. Neuromuscular Disorders of Infancy, Childhood and Adolescence: A Clinician's Approach. Vol. 2. San Diego, CA: Academic Press; 2015. pp. 551-592

[27] Bello L, Morgenroth LP, Gordish-Dressman H, Hoffman EP, McDonald CM, Cirak S, et al. DMD genotypes and loss of ambulation in the CINRG Duchenne natural history study. Neurology. 2016;**87**(4):401-409

[28] Nigro G, Comi LI, Politano L, Bain RJ. The incidence and evolution of cardiomyopathy in Duchenne muscular dystrophy. International Journal of Cardiology. 1990;**26**:271-277

[29] Ricotti V, Mandy WP, Scoto M, Pane M, Deconinck N, Messina S, et al. Neurodevelopmental, emotional, and behavioural problems in Duchenne muscular dystrophy in relation to underlying dystrophin gene mutations. Developmental Medicine and Child Neurology. 2016;**58**:77-84

[30] Tawil R, Van Der Maarel SM. Facioscapulohumeral muscular dystrophy. Muscle & Nerve. 2006; **34**(1):1-15

[31] Banihani R, Smile S, Yoon G, Dupuis A, Mosleh M, Snider A, et al. Cognitive and neurobehavioral profile in boys with Duchenne muscular dystrophy. Journal of Child Neurology. 2015;**30**: 1472-1482

[32] Statland J, Tawil R. Facioscapulohumeral muscular dystrophy. Neurologic Clinics. 2014; **32**(3):721-728

[33] Lilleng H, Abeler K, Johnsen SH, et al. Variation of serum creatine kinase

(CK) levels and prevalence of persistent hyperCKemia in a Norwegian normal population. The Tromsø study. Neuromuscular Disorders. 2011;**21**: 494-500

[34] Koch AJ, Pereira R, Machado M. The creatine kinase response to resistance exercise. Journal of Musculoskeletal & Neuronal Interactions. 2014;**14**(1):68-77

[35] Kim EY. Correlation of serum Creatine kinase level with pulmonary function in Duchenne muscular dystrophy. Annals of Rehabilitation Medicine. 2017;**41**(2):306-312

[36] Swaminathan B, Shubha GN, Shubha D, Murthy AR, Kiran Kumar HB, Shylashree S, et al. Duchenne muscular dystrophy: A clinical, histopathological and genetic study at a neurology tertiary care center in southern India. Neurology India. 2009; **57**:734-738

[37] Love DR, Davies KE. Duchenne muscular dystrophy: The gene and the protein. Molecular Biology & Medicine. 1989;**6**(1):7-17

[38] Wattjes MP, Kley RA, Fischer D. Neuromuscular imaging in inherited muscle diseases. European Radiology. 2010;**20**(10):2447-2460

[39] Guiraud S, Aartsma-Rus A, Vieira NM, Davies KE, van Ommen GJ, Kunkel LM. The pathogenesis and therapy of muscular dystrophies. Annual Review of Genomics and Human Genetics. 2015; **16**:281-308

[40] Charlton R, Henderson M, Richards J, Hudson J, Straub V, Bushby K, et al. Immunohistochemical analysis of calpain 3: Advantages and limitations in diagnosing LGMD2A. Neuromuscular Disorders. 2009;**19**:449-457

[41] Moghadam-Kia S, Oddis CV, Aggarwal R. Approach to asymptomatic creatine kinase activation. Cleveland Clinic Journal of Medicine. 2016;**83**: 37-42

[42] Dubowitz V, Sewry CA, Oldfors A. Immunohistochemistry and immunoblotting. In: Dubowitz V, Sewry CA, Oldfors A, editors. Muscle Biopsy: A Practical Approach. 4th ed. Saunders: Elsevier; 2013. pp. 164-212

[43] Koenig M, Hoffman EP, Bertelson CJ, Monaco AP, Feener C, Kunkel LM. Complete cloning of the Duchenne muscular dystrophy (DMD) cDNA and preliminary genomic organization of the DMD gene in normal and affected individuals. Cell. 1987;**50**:509-517

[44] Ervasti JM, Campbell KP. A role for the dystrophin glycoprotein complex as a transmembrane linker between laminin and actin. The Journal of Cell Biology. 1993;**122**(4):809-823

[45] Vainzof M, Zatz M. Protein defects in neuromuscular diseases. Brazilian Journal of Medical and Biological Research. 2003;**36**:543-555

[46] Zatz M, Vainzof M, Passos-Bueno MR. Limb-girdle muscular dystrophy: One gene with different phenotypes, one phenotype with different genes. Current Opinion in Neurology. 2000; **13**(5):511-517

[47] Bushby K. Report on the 12th ENMC sponsored international workshop—The "limb-girdle" muscular dystrophies. Neuromuscular Disorders. 1992;**2**(1):3-5

[48] Rando T. The dystrophin-glycoprotein complex, cellular signalling, and the regulation of cell survival in the muscular dystrophies. Muscle & Nerve. 2001;**24**:1575

[49] Tews DS, Goebel HH. Diagnostic immunohistochemistry in neuromuscular disorders. Histopathology. 2005;**46**(1):1-23

[50] Pearce M, Blake DJ, Tinsley JM, Byth BC, Campbell L, Monaco AP, et al. The utrophin and dystrophin genes share similarities in genomic structure. Human Molecular Genetics. 1993;**2**(11):1765-1772

[51] Nguyen TM, Ellis JM, Love DR, Davies KE, Gatter KC, Dickson G, et al. Localization of the DMDL gene-encoded dystrophin-related protein using a panel of nineteen monoclonal antibodies: Presence at neuromuscular junctions, in the sarcolemma of dystrophic skeletal muscle, in vascular and other smooth muscles, and in proliferating brain cell lines. The Journal of Cell Biology. 1991; **115**(6):1695-1700

[52] Guiraud S et al. Identification of serum protein biomarkers for utrophin based DMD therapy. Scientific Reports. 2017;7:43697. DOI: 10.1038/srep43697

[53] Dennis CL, Tinsley JM, Deconinck AE, Davies KE. Molecular and functional analysis of the utrophin promoter. Nucleic Acids Research. 1996; **24**(9):1646-1652

[54] Clerk A, Morris GE, Dubowitz V, Davies KE, Sewry CA. Dystrophin-related protein, utrophin, in normal and dystrophic human fetal skeletal muscle. The Histochemical Journal. 1993;**25**(8): 554-561

[55] Bartoli M, Ne'gre P, Wein N, Bourgeois P, Pecheux C, Levy N, et al. Validation of comparative genomic hybridization arrays for the detection of genomic rearrangements of the calpain-3 and dysferlin genes. Clinical Genetics. 2012;**81**:99-101

[56] Lo HP, Cooper ST, et al. Limb-girdle muscular dystrophy: Diagnostic evaluation, frequency and clues to pathogenesis. Neuromuscular Disorders. 2008;**18**(1):34-44

[57] Dubowitz V. Steroids in Duchenne dystrophy. Neuromuscular Disorders. 2013;**23**(7):527-528

[58] Towbin H, Staehelin T, Gordon J. Electrophoretic transfer of proteins from polyacrylamide gels to nitrocellulose sheets: Procedure and some applications. Proceedings of the National Academy of Sciences of the United States of America. 1979;**76**(9): 4350-4354

[59] Burnette WN. Western blotting: Electrophoretic transfer of proteins from sodium dodecyl sulfate-polyacrylamide gels to unmodified nitrocellulose and radiographic detection with antibody and radioiodinated protein a. Analytical Biochemistry. 1981;**112**(2):195-203

[60] Harding A. Not your PI's Western blot. Science. 2013;**339**(6123):1100-1102

[61] Martinez-Flores K, Salazar-Anzures AT, Fernandez-Torres J, Pineda C, Aguilar-Gonzales CA, Lopez-Reyes A. Western blot: A tool in the biomedical field. Investigación en Discapacidad. 2017;**6**(3):128-137

[62] Cooper ST, Lo HP, et al. Single section Western blot: Improving the molecular diagnosis of the muscular dystrophies. Neurology. 2003;**61**(1): 93-97

[63] Anderson LV, Davison K. Multiplex Western blotting system for the analysis of muscular dystrophy proteins. The American Journal of Pathology. 1999; **154**(4):1017-1022

[64] Gaina G, Manole E, Bordea C, Ionica E. Analysis of muscle Calpain3 in LGMDA2A, Studia Universitatis "Vasile Goldis" Arad. Life Sciences Series. 2008; **18**:181-186

[65] Gaina G, Manole E, Bordea C, Mihalcea A, Ionica E. Muscular dystrophies proteins evaluation by western blot and immunofluorescence. Romanian Biotechnological Letters. 2008;**13**(3):3729-3736

[66] Leturcq F, Kaplan JC. Molecular bases of dystrophinopathies. Journal de la Société de Biologie. 2005;**199**(1):5-11

[67] Menezes MP, Waddell LB, et al. The importance and challenge of making an early diagnosis in LMNA-related muscular dystrophy. Neurology. 2012; **78**(16):1258-1263

[68] Chamberlain JS, Gibbs RA, Ranier JE, Nguyen PN, Caskey CT. Multiplex PCR for the diagnosis of DMD. In: Innis MA, Gelfand DH, Sninski J, White T, editors. PCR Protocols: A Guide Methods and Applications. San Diego: Academic Press; 1990. pp. 272-281

[69] Beggs AH, Koenig M, Boyce FM, et al. Detection of 98% of DMD/BMD gene deletions by polymerase chain reaction. Human Genetics. 1990;**86**: 45-48

[70] Abbs S, Yau S, Clark S, Mathew CG. A convenient multiplex PCR system for the detection of dystrophin gene deletions: A comparative analysis with cDNA hybridization shows mistyping by both methods. Journal of Medical Genetics. 1991;**28**(5):304-311

[71] Schouten JP et al. Relative quantification of 40 nucleic acid sequences by multiplex ligation-dependent probe amplification. Nucleic Acids Research. 2002;**30**:e57

[72] Abbs S, Tuffery-Giraud S, Bakker E, Ferlini A, Sejersen T, Mueller CR. Best practice guidelines on molecular diagnostics in Duchenne/Becker muscular dystrophies. Neuromuscular Disorders. 2010;**20**(6):422-430

[73] van Eijk R, Eilers PHC, Natté R, Cleton-Jansen A-M, Morreau H, van Wezel R, et al. MLPAinter for MLPA interpretation: An integrated approach for the analysis, visualisation and data management of multiplex ligation-dependent probe Amplificatio. BMC Bioinformatics. 2010;**11**:67

[74] Jankowski S, Currie-Fraser E, Xu L, Coffa J. Multiplex ligation-dependent probe amplification analysis on capillary electrophoresis instruments for a rapid gene copy number study. Journal of Biomolecular Techniques. 2008;**19**(4): 238-243

[75] Wittwer CT, Herrmann MG, Moss AA, Rasmussen RP. Continuous fluorescence monitoring of rapid cycle DNA amplification. BioTechniques. 2013;**54**(6):314-320

[76] Wittwer CT, Reed GH, Gundry CN, Vandersteen JG, Pryor RJ. High-resolution genotyping by amplicon melting analysis using LCGreen. Clinical Chemistry. 2003;**49**:853-860

[77] Al Momani R, Van Der Stoep N, Bakker E, Den Dunnen JT, Breuning MH, Ginjaar HB. Rapid and cost effective detection of small mutations in the DMD gene by high resolution melting curve analysis. Neuromuscular Disorders. 2009;**19**(6):383-390

[78] Vossen HAM, Roos AEA, den Dunnen JT. High-resolution melting analysis (HRMA)—More than just sequence variant screening. Human Mutation. 2009;**30**:1-7

[79] Porreca GJ. Genome sequencing on nanoballs. Nature Biotechnology. 2010; **28**(1):43-44

[80] Hall N. Advanced sequencing technologies and their wider impact in microbiology. The Journal of Experimental Biology. 2007;**210**(Pt 9): 1518-1525

[81] Pegoraro E, Hoffman EP. Limb-girdle muscular dystrophy overview. In: Pagon RA, Adam MP, Bird TD, Dolan CR, Fong CT, Stephens K, editors. Gene reviews. Seattle, WA, USA: University of Washington; 1993

[82] Roberts RG, Bobrow M, Bentley DR. Point mutations in the dystrophin gene.

Proceedings of the National Academy of Sciences of the United States of America. 1992;**89**:2331-2335

[83] Janssen B, Hartmann C, et al. MLPA analysis for the detection of deletions, duplications and complex rearrangements in the dystrophin gene: Potential and pitfalls. Neurogenetics. 2005;**6**(1):29-35

[84] Schwartz M, Duno M. Improved molecular diagnosis of dystrophin gene mutations using the multiplex ligation-dependent probe amplification method. Genetic Testing. 2004;**8**(4):361-367

[85] Lalic T, Vossen RH, et al. Deletion and duplication screening in the DMD gene using MLPA. European Journal of Human Genetics. 2005; **13**(11):1231-1234

[86] Wu B, Wang L, Dong T, J1 J, Lu Y, Wu H, et al. Identification of a novel DMD duplication identified by a combination of MLPA and targeted exome sequencing. Molecular Cytogenetics. 2017;**23, 10**:8-14

[87] Monaco AP, Bertelson CJ, Liechti-Gallati S, Moser H, Kunkel LM. An explanation for the phenotypic differences between patients bearing partial deletions of the DMD locus. Genomics. 1988;**2**(1):90-95

[88] Aartsma-Rus A, Van Deutekom JC, Fokkema IF, Van Ommen GJ, Den Dunnen JT. Entries in the Leiden Duchenne muscular dystrophy mutation database: An overview of mutation types and paradoxical cases that confirm the reading frame rule. Muscle and NerveMuscle Nerve. 2006; **34**:135-144

[89] Flanigan KM, von Niederhausern A, Dunn DM, Alder J, Mendell JR, Weiss RB. Rapid direct sequence analysis of the dystrophin gene. American Journal of Human Genetics. 2003;**72**:931-939

[90] White S, Kalf M, Liu Q, Villerius M, et al. Comprehensive detection of genomic duplications and deletions in the DMD gene, by use of multiplex amplifiable probe hybridization. American Journal of Human Genetics. 2002;**71**:365-374

[91] Ashton EJ, Yau SC, Deans ZC, Abbs SJ. Simultaneous mutation scanning for gross deletions, duplications and point mutations in the DMD gene. European Journal of Human Genetics. 2008;**16**: 53-61

[92] Nigro V, Savarese M. Genetic basis of limb-girdle muscular dystrophies: The 2014 update. Acta Myologica. 2014; **33**(1):1-12

[93] Sarkozy A, Scoto M, Muntoni F, Domingos J. Dystrophinopathies and limb-girdle muscular dystrophies. Neuropediatrics. 2017;**48**(04):262-272

[94] Kaplan JC, Hamroun D. The 2014 version of the gene table of monogenic neuromuscular disorders (nuclear genome). Neuromuscular Disorders. 2013;**23**(12):1081-1111

[95] Murphy AP, Straub V. The classification, natural history and treatment of the limb girdle muscular dystrophies. Journal of Neuromuscular Diseases. 2015;**2**(s2):S7-S19

[96] Ghaoui R, Cooper ST, Monkol L. Use of whole-exome sequencing for diagnosis of limb-girdle muscular dystrophy: Outcomes and lessons learned. JAMA Neurology. 2015;**72**(12): 1424-1443

[97] Dubowitz V, Sewery C, Lane R. Muscle Biopsy:A Practical Approach. 3th ed. London, UK: Saunders Elsevier; 2007. p. 611

[98] Bovolenta M, Neri M, Ferlini A. novel custom high density-comparative genomic hybridization array detects common rearrangements as well as deep

intronic mutations in dystrophinopathies. BMC Genomics. 2008;**9**:572

[99] Kolski HK, Hawkins C, Zatz M, de Paula F, Biggar D, Alman B, et al. Diagnosis of limb-girdle muscular dystrophy 2A by immunohistochemical techniques. Neuropathology. 2008; **28**(3):264-268

[100] Groen EJ, Charlton R, Barresi R, Anderson LV, Eagle M, Hudson J, et al. Analysis of the UK diagnostic strategy for limb girdle muscular dystrophy 2A. Brain. 2007;**130**:3237-3249

[101] Lanzillo R, Aurino S, Fanin M, Aguennoz M, Vitale F, Fiorillo C, et al. Santoro early onset calpainopathy with normal non-functional calpain 3 level. Developmental Medicine and Child Neurology. 2006;**48**(4):304-306

[102] Fanin M, Nascimbeni A, Fulizio L, Trevisan CP, Meznaric-Petrusa M, Angelini C. Loss of calpain-3 autocatalytic activity in LGMD2A patients with normal protein expression. The American Journal of Pathology. 2003;**163**:1929-1933

[103] Fanin M, Nascimbeni AC, Angelini C. Muscle protein analysis in the detection of heterozygotes for recessive limb girdle muscular dystrophy typ. 2B and 2E. Neuromuscular Disorders. 2006;**16**:792-799

Section 3

Muscular Dystrophy and Central Nervous System

Chapter 3

Cognitive Function and Quality of Life of Muscular Dystrophy

Yukihiko Ueda

Abstract

Duchenne muscular dystrophy and myotonic dystrophy are genetic, progressive muscle diseases. These muscular dystrophies, which are currently incurable, cause muscle wasting or muscle weakness and decrease patients' quality of life. In addition to muscular impairments, cognitive impairments are also reported in both Duchenne muscular dystrophy and myotonic dystrophy. Cognitive impairments in each type of muscular dystrophy are different and closely related to psychosocial variables and the quality of life of the patients. We reviewed the features of cognitive functions in each type of muscular dystrophy and their correlations with the quality of life of patients. Based on the findings, we have suggested effective interventions for improving the quality of life of muscular dystrophy patients.

Keywords: Duchenne muscular dystrophy, myotonic dystrophy, quality of life, cognitive function

1. Introduction

Muscular dystrophy is a genetic, progressive disease of the muscles with several clinical forms, all of which have an early onset and are incurable with current medical technology. These diseases severely decrease motor functions and make it difficult to live an independent social life or engage in an occupation. In this decade, the life span of muscular dystrophy patients has improved considerably as a result of improvements to ventilators. Therefore, it has become necessary to help patients maintain their quality of life (QOL) throughout the life span. Furthermore, muscular dystrophy causes not only physical impairments but also cognitive impairments [1]. Such cognitive impairments are associated with difficulties in communicating with medical workers and family members and also affect medical compliance and the QOL.

2. QOL of patients with muscular dystrophy

Muscular dystrophy has an early onset, and thereafter body functions decrease progressively beginning with a decrease in motor functions that require the use of a wheelchair to maintain mobility and a decrease in the breathing function that require a ventilator to maintain breathing, which makes the patients bedridden. As a result, the patients' behavior repertoire becomes severely restricted, and they require considerable assistance. Netterlund et al. investigated activities of daily living (ADL) and the QOL of 45 people (mean age 44 years) with muscular dystrophy [2] and reported that all the sampled patients were living at home. The QOL was assessed by the Sickness Impact Scale (SIP) and the Psychosocial Well-Being Questionnaire, which indicated that their disability and dependence on others increased, whereas ADL decreased during the previous 5 years. Moreover, the patients' QOL and life satisfaction also decreased. Boström and Ahlström investigated 46 people with muscular dystrophy through interviews using a qualitative research approach for 10 years [3]. They reported that nearly all muscular dystrophy patients had decreasing functions such as limited mobility, increasing fatigue, and feebleness, accompanied by psychological distress. Moreover, if there is a difficulty in securing assistance for patients to continue living in their homes, they must live in recuperation wards.

Ueda et al. [4] investigated the QOL of 50 inpatients with muscular dystrophy. The QOL was assessed by the World Health Organization-Quality of Life 26 (WHO-26). Results indicated that the mean QOL score (SD) of patients with muscular dystrophy was 2.96 (0.34), which was significantly lower than the general Japanese population (mean 3.75) or patients with cancer (mean 3.3). The results of the comparison between patients' conditions indicated that those who could move by using a wheelchair had higher QOL scores than those who were bedridden. The QOL score of patients that had throat surgery was higher than those who had no surgery. The comparison between clinical types indicated that the QOL in myotonic dystrophy was significantly lower than limb girdle-type muscular dystrophy or Fukuyama-type congenital muscular dystrophy. They also investigated factors that could affect the QOL of patients with muscular dystrophy, including age, gender, clinical type, duration of the diseases, throat surgery, duration from throat surgery, functional independence (Barthel Index), use of a ventilator, use of a wheelchair, use of a computer, the frequency of family visits, and participation in activities. The results of categorical regression analysis ($R^2 = 0.671$, $R^2 = 0.400$, $F = 2.479$, $P < 0.05$) showed that only the use of a computer influenced the QOL ($\beta = 0.598$). These results suggest that using a computer could be an effective method of maintaining or improving the QOL of muscular dystrophy inpatients, with deteriorated body functions and limited activities due to the progression of the disease.

3. Profile of cognitive functions in Duchenne muscular dystrophy

Duchenne muscular dystrophy (DMD) is a genetic disease of the muscles caused by deficits in the dystrophin-glycoprotein complex (DGC). The loss of dystrophin is associated with a complex set of physiological and anatomical adaptations that are known contributors to the cognitive deficits observed in patients with DMD and related disorders. Some studies have indicated disordered CNS architecture, abnormalities in dendrites, and loss of neurons in boys with DMD [5]. These boys show EEG abnormalities [5], and the prevalence of epilepsy is higher in DMD (6.3%) than the general population [6]. Studies of CT [7] and MRI [8] have indicated brain atrophy in patients with DMD. These studies suggest that functional and morphological abnormalities are affected by the absence of dystrophins.

Several studies have assessed the intellectual functioning of boys with DMD and reported mean IQs that are approximately one standard deviation lower than the general population [9–12]. Also, boys with DMD have lower verbal IQs (VIQ) than performance IQs (PIQ) [10, 13–16]. Furthermore, Hinton et al. [17] indicated that boys with DMD did poorly on Story Recall, Digit Span, and Auditory Comprehension compared to unaffected siblings. They concluded that verbal working memory was impaired selectively. Moreover, sequential processing ability is more impaired than simultaneous processing ability in boys with DMD [14, 18].

Cotton [19] reported that the boys with DMD had a mean full-scale IQ (FIQ) and a PIQ score of approximately 80 based on a meta-analysis of 1224 boys with DMD. However, the mean VIQ scores improved with age, particularly in the verbal subscales: Information, Similarities, Arithmetic, Comprehension, and Digit Span. Moreover, there were less deficits in older age groups in abilities of logical verbal abstract reasoning, language development, and arithmetic. They suggested the need to adopt more specific and directed neuropsychological assessments to further delineate age-related cognitive changes in DMD populations [19].

3.1 Cognitive functions in adults with DMD

Ueda et al. [20] conducted a study using a wide range of neuropsychological assessment instruments to investigate whether the cognitive weaknesses remain in adult patients with DMD.

Fifteen inpatients and outpatients with DMD (mean age = 30.4 years, age range = 19–44 years) participated in the study. Twenty-four subscales of the Wechsler Adult Intelligence Scale-III (WAIS-III), the Clinical Assessment for Attention (CAT) [21], and the Wechsler Memory Scale (WMS-R) were used for the assessment. The assessment instruments were:

- Ten WAIS-III subscales: (1) Picture Completion, (2) Vocabulary, (3) Similarities, (4) Arithmetic, (5) Matrix Reasoning, (6) Information, (7) Comprehension, (8) Symbol Search, (9) Letter-Number Sequencing, and (10) Digit Span

- Seven subscales of CAT: (11) Auditory Detection, (12) Symbol Digit Modalities, (13) Memory Updating (3 span), (14) Memory Updating (4 span), (15) Paced Auditory Serial Addition Test (PASAT; 2 sec.), (16) PASAT (1 sec.), and (17) Position Stroop

- Seven subscales of WMS-R: (18) Logical Memory, (19) Visual Paired Association, (20) Verbal Paired Associate, (21) Figural Memory, (22) Delayed Logical Memory, (23) Delayed Visual Paired Association, and (24) Delayed Verbal Paired Associates

All assessment instruments were standardized for use in Japan. Therefore, the Z test was used to compare the scores of DMD patients on the 24 subscales with the normal population.

The mean and SD of WAIS-III in DMD adults patients (**Figure 1**), Picture Completion (M = 6.20, SD = 2.86), Arithmetic (M = 5.80, SD = 1.97), Matrix Reasoning (M = 7.47, SD = 3.74), Symbol Search (M = 6.20, SD = 3.84), Letter-Number Sequencing (M = 6.97, SD = 4.64), and Digit Span (M = 7.33, SD = 2.23) were significantly deficient ($p < .01$) compared to the normal population (M = 10, SD = 3). However, there were no significant differences in Vocabulary (M = 8.80, SD = 3.28), Similarities (M = 8.80, SD = 4.31), Information (M = 8.93, SD = 3.08), and Comprehension (M = 9.33, SD = 4.61). The mean FIQ of adult patients with DMD was 87.4 (SD = 15.96, range = 61–109), which was estimated by dyadic short forms of WAIS-III [22, 23].

On the CAT, they were significantly deficient in all subscales (**Figure 2**): Symbol Digit Modalities (M = 42.5, SD = 12.5), Auditory Detection (M = 84.2, SD = 18.8), Memory Updating 3 span (M = 79.2, SD = 25.9), Memory Updating (4 span) (M = 51.4, SD = 30.4), PASAT (2 sec.) (M = 37.2, SD = 30.5), PASAT(1 sec.) (M = 17.4, SD = 16.1), and Position Stroop (M = 97.1, SD = 3.3). In addition, the total Response Time for Position Stroop of patients group (M = 163.0, SD = 75.5) was significantly longer than the normal population.

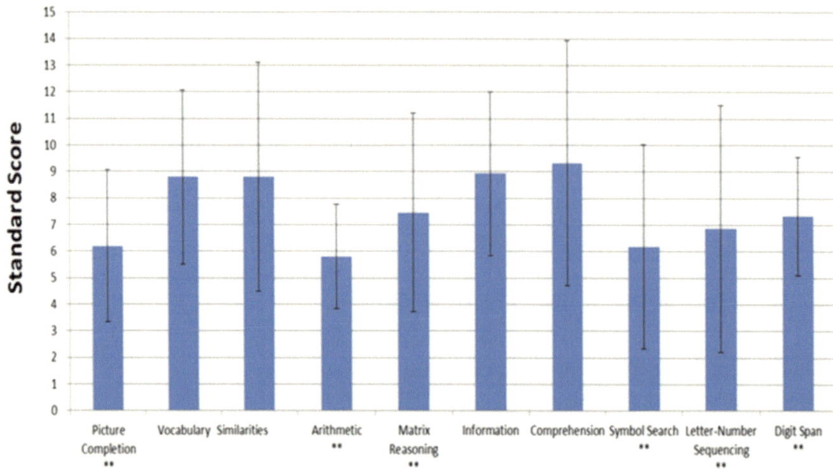

Figure 1.
*Comparison between DMD sample (N = 15) and normal population for WAIS-III. Means and SDs for standard scores are shown. The mean and SD for the normal population are 10 and 3. **p < .01. Ueda et al. [4].*

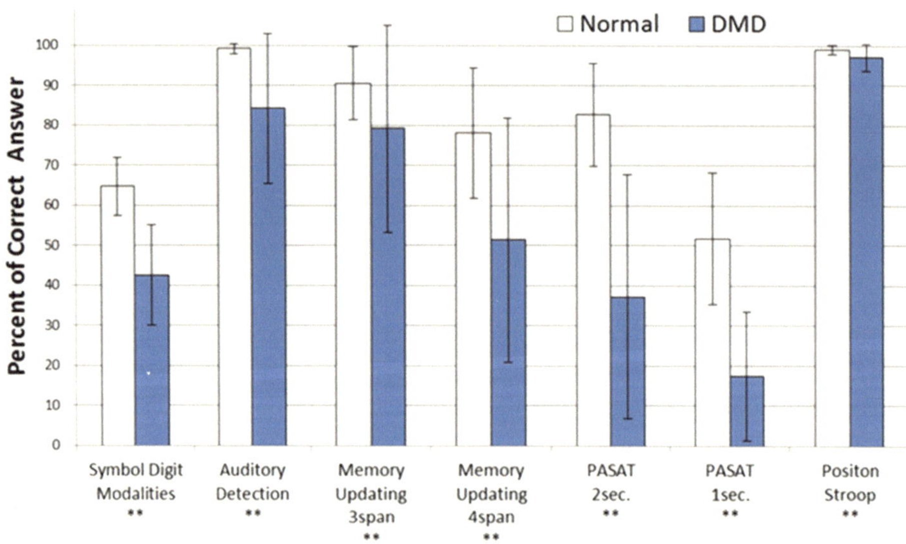

Figure 2.
*Comparison between DMD sample (N = 15) and normal population for CAT. Means and SDs for percentage of correct answers are shown. **p < .01. Ueda et al. [4].*

On the WMS-R, Logical Memory (M = 18.3, SD = 13.1) and Delayed Logical Memory (M = 15.8, SD = 11.7, Z = 2.495, $p < .01$) were significantly lower. However, there were no significant differences between patient group and normal population in other subscales: Visual Paired Association (M = 14.6, SD = 4.1), Verbal Paired Associates (M = 19.3, SD = 5.4), Figural Memory (M = 7.6, SD = 2.0), Delayed Visual Paired Association (M = 5.7, SD = 0.8), and Delayed Verbal Paired Association (M = 7.5, SD = 1.1) (**Figure 3**).

These results indicate that specific cognitive functions of adults with DMD are deficient compared to the normal population. In particular, the ability to sequentially process auditory information was reduced in attention and memory. On the other hand, cognitive abilities that do not require sequential processing were not impaired, suggesting that adults with DMD remain relatively weak in sequential auditory information processing. Moreover, tests of visual information processing showed impairments. These findings suggest that sequential visual information

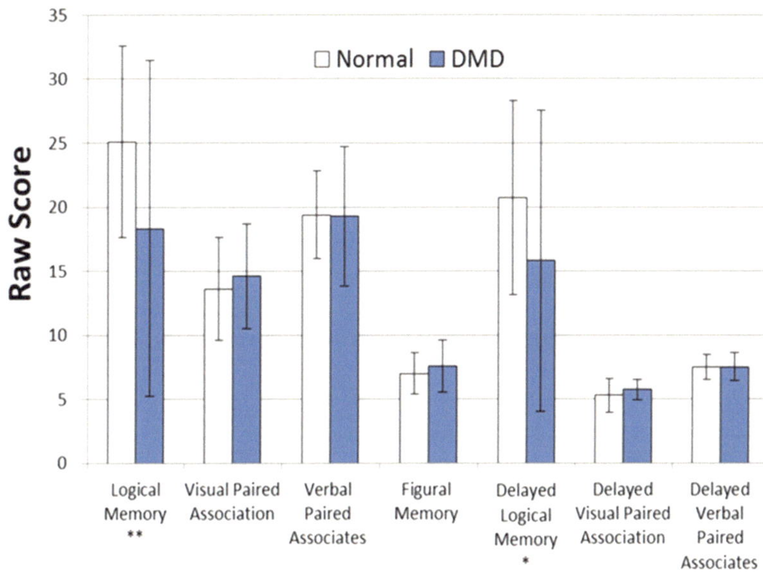

Figure 3.
*Comparison between DMD sample (N = 15) and normal population for WMS-R. Raw means and SDs are shown. *p < .05, **p < .01. Ueda et al. [4].*

processing involving alterations of attention and processing speeds were weak in adult patients with DMD. The weaknesses of cognitive functions were maintained without improvement in adults with DMD. It suggests that these deficits are not caused by environmental factors but represent organic impairments.

Taylor et al. [24] reported differences in neuropsychological profiles of DMD patients and then postulated that these differences are caused by the affected number and type of CNS-expressed isoforms. The site of DMD mutation and the extent of the cognitive deficits are related to each other distinctly. The best model for this phenomenon was that mutations affecting exons 45 to 50 are mainly mutations of coding exons. This effect is restricted to Dp260 and Dp427. In the case of mutations that affected the coding regions of the CNS expressing isoforms Dp140pc and Dp71 are clustered together, there was a significant difference in the degree of cognitive disability. Mutations affecting the Dp140 isoforms affected FIQ less than mutations affecting the Dp140 promoter or protein-coding regions [24]. Nevertheless, the relationship between these isoforms and the ability of sequential information processing has not been clarified. Further research is needed to explore the mechanisms underlining cognitive deficits associated with DGC.

Over the past few decades, the prognosis of DMD patients has shown remarkable improvement; however, the improvement of their quality of life still remains as an important task. Compared with ADHD [25], autistic spectrum disorders, and obsessive–compulsive disorders [25, 26], cognitive problems of DMD patients have been discussed. Particularly, the poor facial recognition of DMD patients [27] might have a negative influence on their QOL. A better evaluation of cognitive deficits in DMD patients could improve their relationship with care staff, thereby contributing to better care and improving the QOL.

4. Cognitive functions of myotonic dystrophy type 1

Myotonic dystrophy type 1 (DM1) is a chronic progressive multi-system disorder with autosomal dominant inheritance. This disorder is caused by a cytosine-thymine-guanine (CTG) repeat expansion in the protein kinase (DMPK) gene [28], resulting in cognitive and psychiatric dysfunctions that have a significant impact on the QOL [29, 30].

Okkersen et al. [31], based on a systematic review and meta-analysis, demonstrated that DM1 patients have significant deficits in all cognitive domains compared to controls. Effect sizes were large (−.76–−1.01) for global cognition, intelligence, visual memory, visuospatial perception, visuoconstruction, psychomotor speed, and social cognition. Moreover, small to medium effect sizes (−.33–−.66) were observed for language, executive functioning, overall and verbal memory, as well as attention.

A few studies have examined the relationship between cognitive impairment and the QOL [30, 32, 33]. However, the majority of these studies did not take all the

Cognitive variable	*n*	Mean	SD	Frequency, %, (95% CI): 1 SD below	Frequency, %, (95% CI): 2 SD below
General cognitive function					
MMSE	60	26.6	3.1		
WAIS-III: Estimated IQ	59	78.8	19.1	63 (51–73)	27 (18–38)
Abstract reasoning					
WAIS-III: Similarities	60	7.7	3.2	52 (40–63)	20 (12–30)
VPTA: Story Telling	57	1.7	2.1	30 (20–41)	7 (2–15)
Attention/working memory					
CAT: Auditory Detection task (%hit)	58	60.4	26.5	79 (69–88)	67 (56–77)
CAT: Auditory Detection task (%correct)	58	82.7	18.9	67 (56–77)	60 (49–71)
CAT: PASAT-2	46	42.2	26	74 (61–84)	41 (29–54)
CAT: Memory Updating 3	57	73.3	22.2	44 (33–56)	30 (20–41)
CAT: Digit Span (backward)	56	4.1	1.2	55 (44–67)	16 (9–26)
CAT: Tapping Span (backward)	57	4.4	1.4	49 (38–61)	9 (4–18)
CAT: Tapping Span (forward)	57	5.7	1.2	26 (17–38)	7 (2–15)
CAT: Digit Span (forward)	56	5.7	1.4	50 (38–62)	5 (1–13)
Executive function					
CAT: Position Stroop test	56	134.3	71.6	86 (76–93)	79 (68–87)
TMT-B	53	220.5	174.5	45 (34–57)	34 (23–46)
FAB	59	15.9	2.0	20 (12–31)	14 (7–23)
WCST: Categories Achieved	55	2.7	2.0	44 (32–56)	11 (5–20)
Phonemic fluency	60	23.7	9.0	40 (29–51)	10 (4–19)
Semantic fluency (animal)	60	17.9	4.6	38 (28–50)	8 (3–17)
Processing speed					
CAT: Visual Cancellation task (Ka)	53	186.6	99.9	96 (89–99)	91 (81–96)
CAT: Symbol Digit Modalities test	56	36.7	14.0	82 (72–90)	54 (42–65)
TMT-A	59	180.9	117.9	66 (55–76)	47 (36–59)
Visuoconstructive ability					
WAIS-III: Block Design	59	4.4	2.5	85 (75–92)	64 (53–75)
VPTA: Copying Figures	56	1.7	1.5	48 (37–60)	48 (37–60)
VPTA: Bisection of Lines	57	1.4	1.5	39 (28–50)	28 (18–39)
VPTA: Copying Flowers	55	2.3	3.3	42 (31–54)	24 (15–35)

Table 1.
Cognitive function of patients with DM1 (Fujino et al. [34]).

domains of cognition into consideration, and they used QOL measures insensitive to specific issues related to DM1.

4.1 Assessment of cognitive function of DM1

Fujino et al. [34] conducted a study of the affected cognitive domains and evaluated the relationship between cognitive functions, psychological factors, and the QOL. Participants (N = 60) were recruited from five hospitals of National Hospital Organization in Japan. The general cognitive functions of the participants were evaluated with the Japanese version of the Mini-Mental State Examination (MMSE), and the estimated IQ was calculated from two subsets (Picture Completion and Information) of WAIS-III. Abstract reasoning was evaluated by using the Similarities subset and the Visual Perceptions Test for Agnosia (VTPA) Story Telling subset [35] in WAIS-III. Attention and working memory were evaluated with CAT subsets (Digit Span [forward, backward], Tapping Span [forward, backward], Auditory Detection task, Memory Updating 3, and PASAT-2. Executive function was evaluated with the Wisconsin Card Sorting Test (WCST), the Frontal Assessment Battery (FAB), the Trail Making Test (TMT)-B, the CAT Position Stroop test, and the semantic and phonemic fluency test. For the assessment of processing speed, TMT-A and 2 CAT subtests (Visual Cancelation task and Symbol Digit Modalities test) were used. For the evaluation of visuoconstructive ability, the WAIS-III Block Design and VPTA subtests (Copying Figures and Flowers, Bisection of Lines) were used. The CAT and VPTA are cognitive functional test batteries, which were developed by the Japan Society for Higher Brain Dysfunction.

As in psychological functioning, the five specific domains were assessed: apathy, depression, excessive daytime sleepiness, fatigue, and social responsiveness. The evaluation tools were Apathy Scale [36], Patients Health Questionnaire-9 (PHQ-9) [37], Epworth Sleepiness Scale (ESS) [38], Multidimensional Fatigue Inventory (MFI) [39], and Social Responsiveness Scale (SRS) [40]. The QOL was estimated with the Muscular Dystrophy Quality of Life Scale (MDQoL) [41] that was developed for Japanese patients with muscular dystrophies including DM1. This scale consists of 10 subscales: Psychological Stability, ADL, Environment, Hope, Activity, Health Relationships, Family, Sexuality, Breathing, and Defecation.

Psychological variable	*n*	Mean	SD	Frequency, %, (95% CI): 1 SD below	Frequency, %, (95% CI): 2 SD below
Apathy					
Apathy Scale	59	18.5	6.4	59 (48–70)	22 (14–33)
Depression					
PHQ-9	60	8	5.5	47 (36–58)	23 (15–34)
Excessive daytime sleepiness					
ESS	59	6.6	4.2	31 (21–42)	5 (1–13)
Fatigue					
MFI	59	64.2	12.0	46 (35–57)	15 (8–25)
Social responsiveness					
SRS	23	56.7	29.7	30 (15–50)	13 (4–30)
QoL (2 factor scores)					
Psychosocial Relationships	57	60.4	17.5		
Physical Functioning and Health	57	62.2	19.0		

Table 2.
Psychological variables and QOL of patients with DM1 (Fujino et al. [34]).

4.2 Cognitive impairments and QOL of DM1

The mean age of the 60 participants with DM1 (35 men and 25 women) was 47.1 (SD = 10.8), and the mean age at the onset of DM1 was 29.0 (SD = 13.2). Moreover, the mean duration of illness was 17.2 years (SD = 11.4). Also, the mean number of CTG repeats was 1132.2 (SD = 1025.2).

The results indicated that most cognitive functions of DM1 patients were lower than the general population (**Table 1**). In particular, more than half of the patients scored 2 SD lower than the general population for attention and working

	Psychosocial Relationships		Physical Function and Health	
Cognitive function	Correlation coefficient	Adjusted *P*-value	Correlation coefficient	Adjusted *P*-value
General cognitive function				
WAIS-III: Estimated IQ	0.27	0.197	0.05	0.850
MMSE	0.16	0.467	0.01	0.975
Abstract reasoning				
WAIS-III: Similarities	0.21	0.313	-0.05	0.857
VPTA: Story Telling	-0.01	0.975	0.02	0.938
Attention/working memory				
CAT: Auditory Detection (%hit)	0.08	0.810	0.03	0.938
CAT: Auditory Detection (%correct)	0.18	0.424	-0.01	0.976
CAT: PASAT-2	0.21	0.389	0.08	0.810
CAT: Tapping Span (backward)	0.30	0.155	0.16	0.467
CAT: Digit Span (backward)	0.29	0.172	0.11	0.606
CAT: Memory Updating 3	0.33	0.081	0.28	0.194
CAT: Digit Span (forward)	0.39*	0.033	0.13	0.589
CAT: Tapping Span (forward)	0.40*	0.030	0.18	0.424
Executive function				
CAT: Position Stroop test	-0.25	0.243	0.08	0.810
TMT-B	-0.27	0.232	-0.15	0.543
FAB	0.20	0.346	0.10	0.654
WCST: Categories Achieved	0.28	0.197	-0.04	0.893
Phonemic fluency	0.14	0.557	-0.16	0.467
Semantic fluency (animal)	0.22	0.306	-0.12	0.589
Processing speed				
CAT: Visual Cancellation task (Ka)	-0.48*	0.006	-0.24	0.275
CAT: Symbol Digit Modalities test	0.22	0.306	0.07	0.810
TMT-A	-0.38*	0.033	-0.06	0.831
Visuoconstructive ability				
WAIS-III: Block Design	0.24	0.243	0.05	0.857
VPTA: Copying Figures	0.03	0.938	0.13	0.589
VPTA: Bisection of Lines	-0.24	0.263	-0.17	0.447
VPTA: Copying lowers	-0.01	0.976	0.07	0.810

**Significant after adjustment using false discovery rate.*

Table 3.
Correlations between cognitive function and QOL (Fujino et al. [34]).

	Psychosocial Relationships		Physical Function and Health	
Psychological measure	Correlation coefficient	Adjusted *P*-value	Correlation coefficient	Adjusted *P*-value
Apathy: Apathy Scale	-0.37*	0.035	-0.20	0.343
Depression: PHQ-9	-0.52*	0.001	-0.65*	<0.001
Excessive daytime sleepiness: ESS	-0.13	0.589	-0.11	0.601
Fatigue: MFI	-0.42*	0.014	-0.55*	<0.001
Social responsiveness: SRS	-0.20	0.589	0.10	0.825

**Significant after adjustment using false discovery rate.*

Table 4.
Correlation between psychological variables and QOL (Fujino et al. [34]).

memory (Auditory Detection task, 67% [hit], 60% [correct]), executive function (Position Stroop test, 79%), processing speed (Visual Cancelation task, 91%, Symbol Digit Modalities test, 54%), and visuoconstructive ability (Block Design, 64%). Although patients were markedly impaired on tasks that assessed complex attentional functions (PASAT-2 and Memory Updating 3), they were not severely affected on those assessing simple attentional functions (Digit Span [forward] and Tapping Span [forward]. Certain patients scored 2 SD higher than the general population on psychological factors including apathy (22%), depression (23%), and fatigue (15%) (**Table 2**).

Factor analysis categorized MDQoL results into Psychosocial relationship factor and Physical functioning and Health factor. The Psychosocial relationship factor was associated with Digit Span (forward, r = 0.39), Tapping Span (forward, r = 0.40), TMT-A (r = −0.38), and Visual Cancelation task (r = −0.48) (**Table 3**). Additionally, the Psychosocial relationship factor was negatively associated with apathy (r = −0.37), depression (r = −0.52), and fatigue (r = −0.42). Physical Functioning and Health factor was negatively associated with depression (r = −0.66) and fatigue (r = −0.55). Apathy was associated with the FAB (r = −0.47), Visual Cancelation (r = 0.46), and Auditory Detection task (r = −0.44) (**Table 4**).

These results demonstrated that patients with DM1 have specific cognitive impairments including executive dysfunctions, processing speed impairments, attentional problems, and visuoconstructive problems. Improved cognitive abilities in attention and working memory, as well as processing speed, were associated with higher QOL, whereas higher apathy, depression, and fatigue were associated with lower QOL. It is possible that apathy mediates the influence of cognitive functions on the QOL, which suggest that the reduction of apathy might lead to better cognitive performance or vice versa [42]. Cognitive assessment can provide useful information for patients, allowing them to plan support in their daily lives. Cognitive interventions might also contribute to improving the QOL of patients with DM1 because neuropsychological rehabilitation and cognitive remediation have been effective in other neurological conditions [43–45].

5. Psychopathological features and personality of DM1 patients

Some studies pointed that depression and fatigue predict psychological and physical QOL in patients with muscular diseases [46, 47]. Additionally, apathy could promote social inhibition and avoidance of social interactions [48]. All of them, in conjunction with each other, lead to the deterioration of the

QOL. Therefore, the psychological interventions for DM1 should incorporate these factors as potential targets for improving patients' QOL.

Minier et al. [49] conducted a systematic literature review of psychopathological features in DM1 and reported that patients with DM1 present mild psychopathological problems, such as interpersonal difficulties, lack of interest, dysphoria, concern about bodily functioning, and hypersensibility. However, they do not present more psychiatric disorders than the general population, except for personality disorders and depression. Moreover, avoidant personality disorder was the most common of several personality disorders among DM1 patients.

5.1 Lack of awareness about the illness

In clinical practice, DM1 patients commonly showed less awareness of the disease distress and its progression. This is named anosognosia or lack of awareness, which can lead to misattributions of symptoms, delay of diagnostic procedures, and low compliance with treatment. The lack of awareness about their illness often is observed in individuals with brain diseases and neurodegenerative disorders, such as Alzheimer's diseases and acquired brain injury. In these disorders, the lack of awareness can be a direct consequence of the underlying pathological process [50]. Research on brain injuries suggests that the prefrontal cortex plays a crucial role in maintaining awareness [51].

Baldanzi et al. [52] conducted a study to estimate the prevalence of disease awareness in 65 adult patients with DM1. The degree of awareness was evaluated by comparing motor impairments using MIRS, patients' complaints about their symptoms, and by comparing INQOL between caregivers. The results indicated that 51.6% of patients were unaware of the disease, and the lack of awareness was most prominent in Independence (52.4%) and Social Relationship (47.6%) domains. Moreover, the lack of awareness was significantly related to failures in cognitive test performance, specifically in the domains of visuospatial memory, cognitive flexibility, and conceptualization. Baldanzi et al. suggested that gaining a better understanding of anosognosia would be useful for the medical management of patients with DM1 and for providing guidance for occupational and social interventions.

6. Interventions

DM1 leads to substantial physical impairments, which in combination with the neuropsychological effects of the condition results in severely restricted social participation. However, there is little evidence for the efficacy of rehabilitative approaches designed to improve health status. Previous studies have demonstrated that fatigue is a highly prevalent, debilitating symptom of DM1 [53, 54], and cognitive behavioral therapy reduces fatigue and increases objective activity, as well as social participation in patients with facioscapulohumeral muscular disease [55]. Therefore, Okkersen et al. [56] conducted a large randomized trial to determine whether cognitive behavioral therapy plus optional graded exercise improved the health status of patients with DM1 compared to standard care alone.

6.1 Cognitive behavioral therapy for the patients with DM1

The study by Okkersen et al. [56] was a large-scale, multicenter, single-blind, randomized trial conducted at four neuromuscular referral centers located in France, Germany, Netherlands, and the UK, which was known as Observational

Prolonged Trial In Myotonic Dystrophy Type 1 to Improve Quality of Life-Standards, a Target Identification Collaboration (OPTIMISTIC). Participants (N = 255) were aged 18 years and older with a confirmed genetic diagnosis of DM1, who were severely fatigued (CIS-fatigue scale, score ≧35) but able to walk independently. They were randomly assigned to either cognitive behavioral therapy plus standard care and optional graded exercise (n = 128) or standard care alone (n = 127). Cognitive behavioral therapy focused on addressing the reduced initiative in the patients, increasing physical activity, optimizing social interactions, regulating sleep–wake patterns, coping with pain, and beliefs about fatigue and DM1. Cognitive behavioral therapy was delivered over a 10-month period in 10–14 sessions based on a manual, by therapists that had extensive training. It was possible to include a graded exercise module that was individually tailored and incorporated moderate-intensity exercises such as walking, cycling, jogging, or dancing for a minimum of 30 minutes, three times a week.

The active-c score of participants in cognitive behavioral therapy increased from a mean (SD) of 61.22 (17.35) at baseline to 63.92 (17.41) at the 10th month. However, the score decreased from 63.00 (17.35) to 60.79 (18.49) in the standard care group. The mean difference between the groups was 3.27 and significant (p = 0.007). As secondary outcomes, the cognitive behavior therapy group showed significant differences in the 6-minute walk test, the fatigue and daytime sleepiness scales, CIS-fatigue, and daily activity levels. Moreover, both groups had decreased scores in the myotonic dystrophy health index and INQOL. However, there was no significant difference between the groups. Also, there were no changes or no differences between the groups on the apathy scale, Stroop-color-word interference, accelerometry for the least active 5 hours, or the Beck Depression Inventory. Based on these results, Okkersen et al. [56] emphasized that cognitive behavioral therapy could increase the capacity for activity and social participation in severely fatigued patients with DM1. This study showed that cognitive behavioral therapy could be one effective intervention for improving the health status of patients with DM1.

7. Conclusion

Cognitive impairments are observed in patients with DMD and DM1. These impairments are caused by gene mutations, especially by CNS-expressed isoforms. These impairments, however, do not encompass every aspect of their intellectual ability. Patients with DMD show deficits in sequential information processing and alterations of attention and processing speed. Moreover, patients with DM1 have weaknesses in executive function, processing speed, attention, and visuoconstructive abilities. These cognitive impairments are related to their psychosocial characteristics, social participation, and the QOL. Especially, apathy, depression, and fatigue are the key factors that deteriorate the QOL of patients with DM1. It is suggested that precisely targeted cognitive assessments and cognitive intervention are necessary to provide them with better care and improve their QOL.

Author details

Yukihiko Ueda
Okinawa International University, Ginowan, Okinawa, Japan

*Address all correspondence to: y.ueda@okiu.ac.jp

References

[1] Orsini M, Andorinho de F, Ferreira A, Damm de Assis A, Magalhães T, Teixeira S, et al. Cognitive impairment in neuromuscular diseases: A systematic review. NI [Internet]. 2018 [cited 10 November 2018];**10**(2). Available from: https://www.pagepress.org/journals/index.php/ni/article/view/7473

[2] Netterlund B et al. Disability, coping and quality of life in individuals with muscular dystrophy: A prospective study over five years. Disability and Rehabilitation. 2000;**22**:776-785

[3] Boström K, Ahlström G. Living with chronic deteriorating disease: The trajectory with muscular dystrophy over ten years. Disability and Rehabilitation. 2004;**26**(17):1388-1398

[4] Ueda Y, Hirayama A, Fukuhara S, Akamine R, Miyagi C, Nakasone M, et al. Quality of life and related factors in inpatients of muscular dystrophy. Sogo Rehabilitation. 2014;**42**(12): 1185-1190. (in Japanese)

[5] Anderson JL, Head SI, Rac C, Morley JW. Brain function in Duchenne muscular dystrophy. Brain. 2002;**125**:4-13

[6] Pane M, Messina S, Bruno C, D'Amico A, Villanova M, Brancalion B, et al. Duchenne muscular dystrophy and epilepsy. Neuromuscular Disorders. 2013;**23**:313-315

[7] Konagaya M, Sakai M, Kuru S, Kato T, Yasuma F, Matsuoka Y. Evaluation of cranial CT findings of patients with muscular dystrophy: With a reference to cerebral vascular disease and cardiac complications(in Japanese). Nō to Shinkei. 1999;**51**:621-626

[8] Doorenweerd N, Straathof CS, Dumas EM, Spitali P, Ginjaar IB, Wokke BH, et al. Reduced cerebral gray matter and altered white matter in boys with Duchenne muscular dystrophy. Annals of Neurology. 2014;**76**:403-411

[9] Bushby KM, Appelton R, Anderson LV, Welch JL, Kelly P, Gardner-Medwin D. Deletion status and intellectual impairment in Duchenne muscular dystrophy. Developmental Medicine and Child Neurology. 1995;**37**:260-269

[10] Michalak M, Opas M. Function of dystrophin and dystrophin associated proteins. Current Opinion in Neurology. 1997;**10**:436-442

[11] Ogasawara A. Downward shift in IQ in persons with Duchenne muscular dystrophy compared to those with spinal muscular atrophy. American Journal of Mental Retardation. 1989;**93**:544-547

[12] Rapaport D, Passos-Bueno MR, Brandao L, Love D, Vainzof M, Zatz M. Apparent association of mental retardation and specific patterns of deletions screened with probes cf56a and cf23a in Duchenne muscular dystrophy. American Journal of Medical Genetics. 1991;**39**:437-441

[13] Billard C, Gillet P, Signoret J, Uicaut E, Bertand P, Fardeau M, et al. Cognitive functions in Duchenne muscular dystrophy: A reappraisal and comparison with spinal muscular atrophy. Neuromuscular Disorders. 1992;**2**:371-378

[14] Dorman C, Hurley AD, D'Avignon J. Language and learning disorders of older boys with Duchenne muscular dystrophy. Developmental Medicine and Child Neurology. 1988;**30**:316-327

[15] Karagan NJ, Zellweger HU. Early verbal disability in children with Duchenne muscular dystrophy. Developmental Medicine and Child Neurology. 1978;**20**:435-441

[16] Marsh GG, Munsat TL. Evidence of early impairment of verbal intelligence in Duchenne muscular dystrophy.

Archives of Disease in Childhood. 1974;**49**:118-122

[17] Hinton VJ, De Vivo DC, Nereo NE, Goldstein E, Stern Y. Selective deficits in verbal working memory associated with a known genetic etiology: The neuropsychological profile of Duchenne muscular dystrophy. Journal of the International Neuropsychological Society. 2001;**7**:45-54. sibling

[18] Ono J, Fujita K. Discrepancy in verbal and performance intellectual ability in children with Duchenne muscular dystrophy (in Japanese). The Japanese Journal of Special Education. 1992;**30**:45-53

[19] Cotton SM, Voudouris NJ, Greenwood KM. Association between intellectual functioning and age in children and young adults with Duchenne muscular dystrophy: Further results from a meta-analysis. Developmental Medicine and Child Neurology. 2005;**47**:257-265

[20] Ueda Y, Suwazono S, Maedo S, Higuchi I. Profile of cognitive function in adults with duchenne muscular dystrophy. Brain and Development. 2017;**39**(3):225-230

[21] Working Group of Brain Function Test, Japan Society for Higher Brain Dysfunction. Clinical Assessment for Attention (CAS) and Spontaneity (CATS) (In Japanese). Tokyo: Shinko Igaku; 2006

[22] Ringe WK, Saine KC, Lacritz LH, Hynan LS, Cullum CM. Dyadic short forms of the Wechsler adult intelligence scale–III. Assessment. 2002;**9**:254-260

[23] Kaufman AS, Ishikuma T, Kaufman-Packer JL. Amazingly short forms of the WAIS-R. Journal of Psychoeducational Assessment. 1991;**9**:4-15

[24] Taylor PJ, Betts GA, Maroulis S, Gilissen C, Pedersen RL, Mowat DR, et al. Dystrophin gene mutation location and the risk of cognitive impairment in Duchenne muscular dystrophy. PLoS One. 2010;**5**:e8803

[25] Pane M, Lombardo ME, Alfieri P, D'Amico A, Bianco F, Vasco G, et al. Attention deficit hyperactivity disorder and cognitive function in Duchenne muscular dystrophy: Phenotype-genotype correlation. The Journal of Pediatrics. 2012;**161**:705-709. e1

[26] Hendriksen JG, Vles JS. Neuropsychiatric disorders in males with Duchenne muscular dystrophy: Frequency rate of attention-deficit hyperactivity disorder (ADHD), autism spectrum disorder, and obsessive-compulsive disorder. Journal of Child Neurology. 2008;**23**:477-481

[27] Hinton VJ, Fee RJ, De Vivo DC, Goldstein E. Poor facial affect recognition among boys with Duchenne muscular dystrophy. Journal of Autism and Developmental Disorders. 2007;**37**:1925-1933

[28] Harper PS. Myotonic Dystrophy. 3rd ed. London: WB Saunders; 2001

[29] Meola G, Sansone V. Cerebral involvement in myotonic dystrophies. Muscle & Nerve. 2007;**36**(3):294-306

[30] Raekocevic-Stojanovic V, Peric S, Madzarevic R, Dobricic V, Ralic V, Ilic V, et al. Significant impact of behavioral and cognitive impairment and quality of life in patients with myotonic dystrophy type 1. Clinical Neurology and Neurosurgery. 2014;**126**:76-81

[31] Okkersen K, Buskes M, Groenewound J, Kessels RPC, Knoop H, Engelen BV, et al. The cognitive profile of myotonic dystrophy type 1: A systematic review and meta-analysis. Cortex. 2017;**95**:143-155

[32] Antonini G, Socia F, Giubilei F, De Carolis A, Gragani F, Morino

S, et al. Health rerated quality of life in myotonic dystrophy type 1 and its relationship with cognitive and emotional functioning. Journal of Rehabilitation Medicine. 2006;**38**:181-185

[33] Sansone VA, Panzeri M, Montanari M, Apolone G, Gandossini S, Rose MR, et al. Italian validation of INQoL, a quality of life questionnaire for adults with muscle diseases. European Journal of Neurology. 2010;**17**:1178-1187

[34] Fujino H, Shingaki H, Suwazono S, Ueda Y, Wada C, Nakayama T, et al. Cognitive impairment and quality of life in patients with myotonic dystrophy type 1. Muscle & Nerve. 2018;**57**(5):742-748

[35] Japan Society for Higher Brain Dysfunction. Visual Perceptions Test for Agnosia: VTPA. Revised. Tokyo: Shinko Igaku Shuppan; 2003

[36] Starkstein SE, Fedoroff JP, Price TR, Leiguarda R, Robinson RG. Apathy following cerebrovascular lesions. Stroke. 1993;**24**:1625-1630

[37] Kroenke K, Spitzer RL, Williams JB. The PHQ-9: Validity of a brief depression severity measure. Journal of General Internal Medicine. 2001;**16**:606-613

[38] Takegami M, Suzukamo Y, Wakita T, Noguchi H, Chin K, Kadotani H, et al. Development of Japanese version of the Epworth sleepiness scale (JESS) based on item response theory. Sleep Medicine. 2009;**10**:556-565

[39] Smets EM, Garssen B, Bonke B, De Haes JC. The multidimensional fatigue inventory (MFI) psychometric qualities of an instrument to assess fatigue. Journal of Psychosomatic Research. 1995;**39**:315-325

[40] Constantino JN, Davis SA, Todd RD, Schindler MK, Gross MM, Brophy SL, et al. Validation of a brief quantitative measure of autistic traits: Comparison of the social responsiveness scale with the autism diagnostic interview-revised. Journal of Autism and Developmental Disorders. 2003;**33**:427-433

[41] Kawai M, Ono M, Yatabe K, Ohya N, Saito T, Sugiyama H, et al. Development of MDQoL-60 for Patients with Muscular Dystrophy. Hasuda, Saitama: Higashisaitama National Hospital; 2005. p. 2005. (in Japanese)

[42] Lohner V, Brooker RI, Hollocks MJ, Morris RG, Markus HS. Apathy, but not depression, is associated with executive dysfunction in cerebral small vessel diseases. PLoS One. 2017;**12**:e0176943

[43] Blunelle-Hamann I, Thivierge S, Simard M. Impact of a cognitive rehabilitation intervention on neuropsychiatric symptoms in mild to moderate Alzheimer's diseases. Neuropsychological Rehabilitation. 2015;**25**:677-707

[44] Edwards JD, Hauser RA, O'Connor MI, Valdes EG, Zesiewicz TA, Uc EY. Randomized trial of cognitive speed of processing training in Parkinson diseases. Neurology. 2013;**81**:1284-1290

[45] Rosti-Otajarvi EM, Hamalainen PI. Neuropsychological rehabilitation for multiple sclerosis. Cochrane Database of Systematic Reviews. 2014:CD009131

[46] Rose MR, Sadjadi R, Weinman J, Akhtar T, Pandya S, Kissel JT, et al. Role of disease severity, illness perceptions, and mood on quality of life in muscle disease. Muscle & Nerve. 2012;**46**:351-359

[47] Kalkman JS, Schillings ML, Zwarts MJ, van Engelen BG, Bleijenberg G. The development of a model of fatigue in neuromuscular disorders: A longitudinal study. Journal of Psychosomatic Research. 2007;**62**:571-579

[48] Meola G, Sansone V, Perani D, Scarone S, Cappa S, Dragoni C, et al. Executive dysfunction and avoidant personality trait in myotonic dystrophy type 1 (DM-1) and in proximal myotonic myopathy (PROMM/ DM-2). Neuromuscular Disorders. 2003;**13**:813-821

[49] Minier L, Lignier B, Bouvet C, Gallais B, Camart N. A review of psychopathology features, personality, and coping in myotonic dystrophy type 1. Journal of Neuromuscular Diseases. 2018;**5**(3):279-294

[50] De Carolis A, Cipollini V, Corigliano V, Comparelli A, Sepe-Monti M, Orzi F, et al. Anosognosia in people with cognitive impairment: Association with cognitive deficits and behavioral disturbances. Dementia and Geriatric Cognitive Disorders Extra. 2015;**5**(1):42-50

[51] Stuss D. Disturbances of self-awareness after frontal system damage. In: Prigatano GP, Schacter DL, editors. Awareness of Deficit after Brain Injury: Clinical and Theoretical Issues. New York: Oxford Press; 1991. pp. 63-83

[52] Baldanzi S, Bevilacqua F, Lorio R, Volpi L, Simoncini C, Petrucci A, et al. Disease awareness in myotonic dystrophy type 1: An observational cross-sectional study. Orphanet Journal of Rare Diseases. 2016;**11**(34). DOI: 10.1186/s13023-016-0417-z

[53] Kalkman JS, Schillings ML, van der Werf SP, et al. Experienced fatigue in facioscapulohumeral dystrophy, myotonic dystrophy, and HMSN-1. Journal of Neurology, Neurosurgery, and Psychiatry. 2015;**76**:1406-1409

[54] Heatwole C, Bode R, Johnson N, et al. Patient-reported impact of symptoms in myotonic dystrophy type 1 (PRISM-1). Neurology. 2012;**79**:348-357

[55] Voet N, Bleijenberg G, Hendriks J, et al. Both aerobic exercise and cognitive-behavioral therapy reduce chronic fatigue in FSHD: An RCT. Neurology. 2014;**83**:1914-1922

[56] Okkersen K, Jimenez-Moreno C, Wenninger S, Daidjf F, Glennon J, Cumming S, et al. cognitive behavioral therapy with optimal graded exercise therapy in patients with severe fatigue with myotonic dystrophy type 1: A multicenter, single-blind, randomized trial. The Lancet Neurology. 2018;**17**(8):671-680

Chapter 4

Electrophysiological Assessment of CNS Abnormalities in Muscular Dystrophy

Stefan M. Golaszewski and Raffaele Nardone

Abstract

Patients affected by muscular dystrophies often show CNS abnormalities. Patients with dystrophinopathies exhibit intellectual disabilities and mental retardation, while subjects with facioscapulohumeral muscular dystrophy (FSHD) often show epilepsy. Dystrophin and associated proteins have important roles in the CNS. Many patients with Duchenne and Becker muscular dystrophies (DMD/BMD) have cognitive impairment, learning disability, and variable degrees of mental retardation in addition to progressive muscular weakness. Unfortunately, the assessment of cortical function with TMS in DMD patients has not been able to delineate a clear picture and has yielded contradictory results. No TMS studies have been performed on BMD patients. Repetitive transcranial magnetic stimulation (rTMS) modulates cortical excitability, possibly by inducing a short-term increase in synaptic efficacy, and can be used to investigate motor cortex excitability in BMD patients. Changes in the size and threshold of motor evoked potentials (MEPs) and cortical silent period (CSP) duration evoked by rTMS delivered in 5 Hz trains of stimuli at suprathreshold intensity can be tested. Impaired muscular function might be partially compensated by an enhancement of motor excitability at the cortical level and/or at α-motoneuron level. TMS may thus offer a reliable means to characterize also important neurophysiologic and pathophysiologic aspects of cortical involvement in muscular dystrophy.

Keywords: transcranial magnetic stimulation, paired-pulse TMS, motor cortical excitability, myopathy, muscular dystrophy

1. Introduction

Muscular dystrophy (MD) is characterized by an absence or disruption of dystrophin and associated proteins with a severe pathology of the skeletal musculature with severe motor disabilities and even premature death of the individual. These proteins do not only have an important function within the skeletal musculature but also within the central nervous system. Thus, patients with muscular dystrophies often suffer from cognitive impairment, learning disability, and variable degrees of mental retardation in addition to progressive muscular weakness [1–3]. Patients with facioscapulohumeral muscular dystrophy (FSHD) are often affected by epilepsy [4, 5]. However, the pathogenetic role played by the absence or disruption of dystrophin on CNS function has not been clarified so far.

Transcranial magnetic stimulation (TMS) is a proper method to assess brain cortical excitability that is disturbed in muscular dystrophies. A TMS assessment of brain cortical function in DMD patients has yielded contradictory results [6]. While Yayla et al. reported no CNS abnormalities and similar motor threshold (MT) values in DMD patients and healthy controls, Di Lazzaro et al. reported a higher MT for magnetic than for electrical stimulation in four DMD patients [7]. Methodological reasons, as well as the small sample size of the latter study, may account for the discrepancies. Because repetitive TMS (rTMS) modulates cortical excitability, possibly by inducing a short-term increase in synaptic efficacy [8], rTMS can be used to investigate motor cortex excitability in humans. Changes in the size and threshold of motor evoked potentials (MEPs) and cortical silent period (CSP) duration evoked by rTMS delivered in 5 Hz trains of stimuli at supra-threshold intensity have been tested by Golaszewski et al. [9]. The main finding of this study was that 5 Hz-rTMS delivered in trains failed to elicit the normal MEP facilitation over the train in a group of Becker Muscular Dystrophy (BMD) patients with mental retardation or borderline mental retardation and BMD patients with normal intelligence and healthy controls did not show any abnormalities in 5 Hz-rTMS MEPs and CSPs. The lack of MEP facilitation in mentally retarded or borderline BMD patients during the 5 Hz-rTMS train of stimuli may thus reflect an altered short-term synaptic enhancement.

With the means of transcranial magnetic stimulation, important neurophysiologic and pathophysiologic aspects of cortical involvement in myopathies can be detected [10, 11]. So far, a few studies applying TMS have detected abnormalities in cortical reactivity and plasticity in MD patients.

2. Electrophysiological markers in muscular dystrophy

2.1 Motor threshold

In a study of Di Lazzaro et al. in a small group of DMD patients and a control group (n = 4), the threshold for evoking MEPs using electrical anodal stimulation was the same. Otherwise, the resting motor threshold (RMT) for a stimulation with a circular magnetic coil at the vertex was higher in the DMD patients [7]. The higher threshold was interpreted as a reduced cortical excitability that may be related to an abnormal synaptic function due to the deficiency of brain synaptic dystrophin. However, in a study about the cortical excitability in Duchenne muscular dystrophy investigating central motor conduction time (CMCT), cortical silent periods, and paired-pulse TMS, there were no statistical differences between a group of DMD children and a group of age-matched control children except lower MEP amplitudes in the DMD children. Compared with a control group of healthy adults, the two children groups showed less short interval intracortical inhibition (SICI) and shorter CSP durations [6]. The difference between the two studies can be explained by the applied different methods, since in the study by Di Lazzaro et al., a circular coil was used and an unusual minimum stimulus intensity that evoked an EMG response of at least 100 μV in 100% of 20 consecutive trials was the accepted resting motor threshold. Besides the small sample size in the study of Di Lazzaro et al. can be an explanation for the difference.

Oliveri et al. found that in patients with myotonic dystrophy, the stimulus threshold intensity did not differ between patients and healthy controls, but the mean cortical motor latency and CMCT were significantly prolonged in the patients compared to the controls. This can be interpreted as a central motor delay and a decreased excitability of motor neurons in the myotonic dystrophy patients [12].

In another study Di Lazzaro et al. [13] found that RMT was slightly increased in patients with FSHD as well as in patients with other muscle diseases such as limb-girdle muscle dystrophy (LGMD) and polymyositis [13]. However, Liepert et al. [14] could not show a significant difference in RMT between a group of patients with different myopathies (including FSHD, LGMD, emerinopathy, adhalinopathy, multicore disease) and a group of control subjects [14].

2.2 Central motor conduction time

As mentioned above Oliveri et al. investigated MEPs elicited by cortical and cervical magnetic stimulation in 10 patients with myotonic dystrophy. While MEP cervical latency, absolute or relative amplitude, and RMT did not differ significantly between patients and controls, the mean cortical motor latency and CMCT were significantly prolonged in the patients compared with 10 healthy controls [12]. This central motor delay can be explained by a decreased motoneuron excitability.

In several further studies, it was found that CMCT was normal in patients with FSHD and LGMD [13, 14] as well as in patients with DMD [6, 7].

2.3 MEP amplitudes/areas

Yayla et al. further described in his study [6] with DMD patients that mean MEP response amplitudes and areas, as well MEP/compound muscle action potential (CMAP) amplitude ratios, had a tendency to be lower than those of a control group, but only the differences in MEP area values reached a statistical significance [6]. An explanation for the reduced amplitude of CMAPs and MEPs could be the muscle damage in the DMD patients. Otherwise, DMD patients showed an increased ratio of the F-wave and the compound motor action potential (F/CMAP ratio), indicative for an increased α-motoneuron excitability. The mean F-wave amplitudes were not significantly different between DMD patients and controls. Therefore, the reason for a higher F/CMAP ratio in the DMD group is difficult to explain. One explanation may be an increased F-wave amplitude in the DMD patients that did not reach statistical significance especially due to their large variability. Another explanation may be the aforementioned low-amplitude CMAPs in DMD patients or an increased motor cortical excitability due to less SICI and shorter CSP durations in DMD patients with regard to healthy adult controls.

In the study of Liepert et al., MEP amplitudes of the first dorsal interosseous (FDI) and the deltoid muscle (DM) were increased in patients with different myopathies compared to controls [14]. The recruitment of a larger group of corticospinal neurons by the TMS pulses due to an increased motor cortical excitability with a consecutive increased activation of the α-motoneuron pool may explain this finding.

Finally, in the study of Oliveri et al., the first MEP study in patients with myotonic dystrophy, the mean MEP amplitudes did not differ between patients and controls [12].

2.4 Intracortical inhibition

In the study of Liepert et al. in myopathy patients with well-defined myopathies, the patients showed a reduction of SICI compared to an age-matched healthy control group [14]. This reduction of SICI was present in both clinically unaffected and affected muscles. In the patients, both MEP amplitudes and α-motoneuron excitability were enhanced, and, thus, it was concluded that excitability in myopathy patients was enhanced at cortical and subcortical levels in order to compensate for the muscle weakness or because of use-dependent plasticity. In all patients irrespective of the type of myopathy, a reduced intracortical inhibition was found. Obviously, this neurobiological mechanism of increased motor cortical excitability for compensation of muscle weakness is independent of a particular muscle pathology in myopathies. However, with regard to the available electrophysiological data, there is no sufficient evidence to conclude that cortical disinhibition is a common feature of myopathies.

In 2004 Di Lazzaro et al. reported significantly reduced SICI in early-onset FSHD patients compared with patients suffering from other muscle diseases (LGMD and polymyositis) and healthy controls. Between polymyositis patients and controls, there was no significant difference in SICI [13].

2.5 TMS and fatigue

During fatiguing muscle exercise, a paired-pulse TMS paradigm can be applied to investigate the central inhibitory and excitatory mechanisms that occur at the motor cortical level. Paired-pulse TMS was already done in patients with multiple sclerosis and in healthy subjects [15, 16]. In a study of Schwenkreis et al., SICI has been applied prior to a fatiguing motor task, immediately post-exercise, and 40 minutes post-exercise in MD patients and patients suffering from fibromyalgia syndrome (FMS) [17]. In the MD and FMS patients, SICI was already reduced pre-exercise. Healthy subjects did not show any pre-exercise SICI decrease but a significant SICI decrease post-exercise. Thus, reduced SICI may be a central compensatory mechanism for peripheral or central fatigue. MD patients may use this neurobiological mechanism of reduced SICI already under baseline conditions, probably due to permanent muscle weakness. Probably due to a ceiling effect, the MD and FMS patients may not be able to further decrease cortical inhibition during the fatiguing exercise. This may be an additional central mechanism to the fatigue in MD and FMS patients. A fatigue syndrome belongs to the typical clinical feature of these patients.

An altered peripheral nerve excitability and reduced SICI at baseline in patients with MD type 1 (DM1) with impaired myoelectric properties (mean power frequency, muscle fiber conduction velocity) have been demonstrated in a study of Boerio et al. [18]. The remaining excitability parameters did not vary post-exercise in patients in contrast to the healthy controls.

In patients with colchicine myopathy with reported fatigue but no significant muscle weakness, Lin et al. investigated central compensatory mechanisms [19]. The patient and control group did not differ in the results. Obviously, there is no change in motor cortical excitability in acquired myopathy due to colchicine, while central reorganization may occur in patients with hereditary myopathy to compensate for muscle weakness.

2.6 Cortical plasticity

Repetitive TMS has also been applied to investigate motor cortex plasticity in patients with Becker muscular dystrophy [9]. The rTMS-induced facilitation of MEPs was significantly reduced in mentally retarded or borderline mentally retarded classified BMD patients when compared with BMD patients with normal intelligence and age-matched healthy controls (see **Figure 1a**). The increase in the duration of the cortical silent periods was similar in both patient groups and controls (see **Figure 1b**). These findings suggest an altered cortical short-term synaptic plasticity in glutamate-dependent excitatory circuits within the motor cortex in BMD patients with intellectual disabilities.

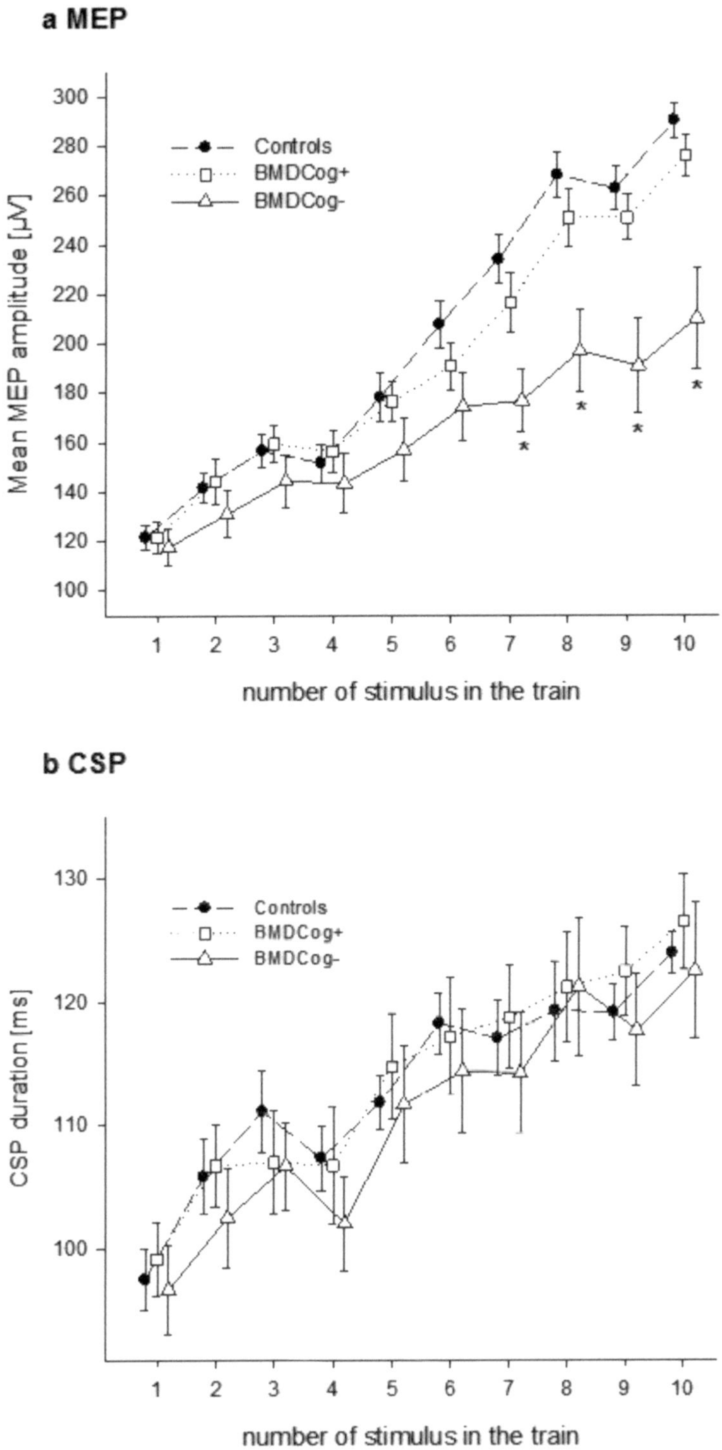

Figure 1.
(a and b) Changes in the size of motor evoked potentials (a) and in the duration of cortical silent period (b) in the FDI muscle during repetitive transcranial magnetic stimulation trains of 10 pulses delivered at 5 Hz in the 6 patients with Becker muscular dystrophy and mental retardation or borderline (BMD-Cog−), the 7 patients with BMD and normal intelligence (BMD-Cog+), and the 10 age-matched healthy subjects (controls). Data are expressed as mean ± SE. Asterisks indicate significant differences ($p < 0.05$, Bonferroni adjusted) between patients and controls.

3. Discussion

The studies reviewed here show that most TMS measurements vary considerably from study to study. The cause of this variability remains unclear, but the methodological problem of TMS and technical factors, including the relatively small sample size in most studies or the difficulty of many patients (especially children) to achieve complete muscle relaxation, can explain this variability. Several TMS studies have provided electrophysiological evidence for abnormal motor cortical excitability and/or plasticity in patients with different myopathies. Applications of TMS to characterize musculoskeletal pathophysiology in patients with myopathies appear to be safe and can be developed in valuable biomarkers.

In a first study of patients with MD, TMS has been reported to have subclinical central motor conduction abnormalities suggesting that the integrity of the corticospinal tract is also affected. This deficiency was considered one of the multisystem manifestations of muscle disease, regardless of muscle pathology [12]. However, these preliminary results were not confirmed by successive studies in other myopathies.

The reviewed TMS studies showed that it is possible to detect changes in motor cortex excitability in myopathy patients. The most important finding is a significant reduction in SICI compared to healthy controls.

In adult patients with various types of myopathies, including FSHD and LGMD, the mechanisms of intracortical inhibition are reduced. This finding has been interpreted as a compensatory mechanism within the central nervous system that helps patients with myopathy to regain muscle power. SICI deficiency in FSHD may be explained by overexpression of the gene encoding the diazepam binding inhibitor (DBI), which is expected to attenuate the effects of GABA on $GABA_A$ receptors by acting on the benzodiazepine binding site [20]. Thus, DBI can determine a reduction in SICI, a phenomenon that depends largely on intracortical $GABA_A$ inhibitory mechanisms. It is interesting to note that a decrease in initial intracortical inhibition may prevent the subsequent use of this compensatory mechanism within the central nervous system in fatiguing muscle exercises as can be seen in healthy subjects [17]. Reduced baseline SICI in MD can be considered compensatory because of peripheral weakness, whereas in fibromyalgia syndrome, reduced SICI should rather be considered as an indicator of primary central disinhibition. Also in DM1 patients, TMS revealed abnormalities in cortical excitability, thus suggesting the occurrence of intracortical dysfunction [18]. These results are consistent with the autopsy and neuroimaging studies showing that dysfunction of the brain can be accompanied by structural changes. As a result, a disturbance of neuronal architecture was detected in the autopsy of the brain [21]. In addition, a three-dimensional magnetic resonance imaging-controlled study demonstrated cerebral parenchymatrophy and hyperintensive lesions of the white matter [22], and PET scans showed a hypoperfusion in the prefrontal, temporal, and parieto-occipital lobes as well as in the basal ganglia, supporting the hypothesis of brain dysfunction in patients with DM1 [23].

In DM1 patients reduced intracortical facilitatory mechanisms (ICF) were found too [18]. Further, CNS excitability properties were markedly altered at the baseline and were not prone to be further impaired after a fatiguing exercise. Adjusting the cortical and neuromuscular features to the initial change may prevent increased fatigue after exercise performed with a maximum voluntary contraction percentage. The authors hypothesized that fatigue in MD patients may be mainly due to peripheral factors related to muscle pathology. Thus, MD patients were probably unable to reach the required force level of 50% of their maximal grip force for enough time to determine a reduction of corticospinal excitability, a marker of central fatigue [24]. This may explain the lack of reduced MEP amplitudes after fatiguing exercise in these patients.

It is interesting to note that central compensatory mechanisms can be observed in patients with hereditary myopathies, whereas a single study on TMS in an acquired colchicine myopathies showed normal corticospinal excitability.

Many patients with dystrophinopathies (DMD and BMD) also suffer from cognitive impairment, learning difficulties, and variable mental retardation in addition to progressive muscle weakness [1–3]. The role played by the absence or disruption of dystrophin within the central nervous system is unclear, and the pathogenic conditions leading to mental retardation in MD patients are still unknown. TMS investigation of cortical function in DMD patients did not delineate a clear picture of motor cortical abnormalities and led even to contradictory results. Yayla et al. did not report any motor cortical abnormalities [6], and Di Lazzaro et al. reported higher MT for magnetic than for electrical stimulation in four DMD patients [7]. As already discussed, methodological reasons, as well as the small sample size of the latter study, may account for these discrepancies.

During 5 Hz-rTMS in BMD patients, MEP facilitation as observed in healthy subjects was reduced in contrast to the above-reported study of Yayla et al. [6, 9]. 5 Hz-rTMS MEP facilitation reflects mechanisms of short-term plasticity within the motor cortex that probably differ from those involved in the paired-pulse TMS facilitation and are likely related to an enhancement in the activity of I-wave generating circuits [25]. Intracortical facilitation in paired-pulse TMS is a complex phenomenon reflecting the activity of still poorly defined cortical circuits independent from those involved in I-wave generation [26].

The results of the study of Golaszewski et al. indicate impaired cortical plasticity in glutamate-dependent excitation circuits in mentally retarded BMD patients consistent with the results of several experimental studies indicating abnormal glutamatergic transmission in muscle diseases caused by mutations within the dystrophin-encoding gene [9]. In particular, the product of the dystrophin gene, dystrophin-71, in glutamate receptor signaling and possibly clustering, appears to be involved [27]. Besides, dystrophin-deficient mdx mice are more resistant to kainic acid-induced seizures but not to GABA antagonist-induced seizures compared with control mice. In the mdx mice, the kainic acid receptor density in the brain was found to be significantly lower than in the control mice, although the density of muscarinic cholinergic receptors, another important neurotransmitter receptor for cognitive function, was normal. The disruption of the dystrophin complex may lead to an instability of kainate-type glutamate receptors on the synaptic membranes with resulting inefficient neurotransmission in DMD patients [28].

It is important to note that the rTMS approach cannot be used to study cortical plasticity in children with DMD because the safety guidelines for the TMS application have been updated in the research and clinical environments [29]. The updated guidelines recommend that children should not be used as subjects for rTMS without compelling clinical reasons. Alternatively, the paired associative stimulation (PAS) technique can be applied in MD children that provide information about different aspects of cortical plasticity. So far, PAS has not yet been applied in myopathy patients and MD children [30]. No study has measured cortical responsiveness or plasticity outside the motor cortex.

Integrated approaches using TMS in conjunction with high-density EEG may reveal altered cortical plasticity and functional connectivity across different neuronal networks, similar to several other neurological and psychiatric disorders.

TMS can also affect brain function during repeated administration. rTMS can modulate cortical excitability and induce long-lasting neuroplastic changes [31, 32]. rTMS has been used for therapeutic purposes in patients with many neurological and psychiatric disorders because it can induce long-term modulation of brain activity in the target brain region and across brain networks via transcranial induction of electrical currents in the brain. rTMS involves mechanisms of synaptic plasticity, and, recently, an association between rTMS-induced aftereffects and the induction of synaptic plasticity has been demonstrated [33]. Since abnormal cortical excitability and neuroplastic changes may play a role in the clinical expression of myopathies (including muscle weakness and fatigue), their modulation by rTMS may have a therapeutic potential. If the abovementioned changes affect motor control, treatment, or rehabilitation, strategies based on these abnormalities can help to improve the outcome of myopathy patients in neurorehabilitation.

In summary, only a few studies have used TMS for the electrophysiological characterization of cortical involvement in neuromuscular diseases. However, TMS may be promising as an electrophysiological biomarker in patients with muscular dystrophy and other myopathies, in identifying potential therapeutic targets and in monitoring the effects of suspected pharmacological applications. Neuromodulation by rTMS may have a therapeutic potential in the future to induce synaptic plasticity as a compensatory neurobiological mechanism for progressive muscle weakness to improve treatment outcome.

Author details

Stefan M. Golaszewski[1,3]* and Raffaele Nardone[1,2,3]

1 Department of Neurology and Neuroscience Institute, Paracelsus Medical University, Salzburg, Austria

2 Department of Neurology, Franz Tappeiner Hospital, Meran, Italy

3 Karl Landsteiner Institute for Neurorehabilitation and Space Neurology, Salzburg, Austria

*Address all correspondence to: s.golaszewski@salk.at

References

[1] Emery AEH. Central nervous system. In: Motulsky AG, editor. Duchenne Muscular Dystrophy. New York: Oxford University Press; 1987. pp. 99-106

[2] Mehler MF. Brain dystrophin, neurogenetics and mental retardation. Brain Research. Brain Research Reviews. 2000;**32**(1):277-307

[3] North KN et al. Cognitive dysfunction as the major presenting feature of Becker's muscular dystrophy. Neurology. 1996;**46**(2):461-465

[4] Grosso S et al. Epilepsy, speech delay, and mental retardation in facioscapulohumeral muscular dystrophy. European Journal of Paediatric Neurology. 2011;**15**(5):456-460

[5] Saito Y et al. Facioscapulohumeral muscular dystrophy with severe mental retardation and epilepsy. Brain and Development. 2007;**29**(4):231-233

[6] Yayla V et al. Cortical excitability in Duchenne muscular dystrophy. Clinical Neurophysiology. 2008;**119**(2):459-465

[7] Di Lazzaro V et al. Functional involvement of cerebral cortex in Duchenne muscular dystrophy. Muscle & Nerve. 1998;**21**(5):662-664

[8] Fisher SA, Fischer TM, Carew TJ. Multiple overlapping processes underlying short-term synaptic enhancement. Trends in Neurosciences. 1997;**20**(4):170-177

[9] Golaszewski S et al. Abnormal short-latency synaptic plasticity in the motor cortex of subjects with Becker muscular dystrophy: A rTMS study. Neuroscience Letters. 2016;**610**:218-222

[10] Hallett M. Transcranial magnetic stimulation and the human brain. Nature. 2000;**406**(6792):147-150

[11] Rossini PM et al. Non-invasive electrical and magnetic stimulation of the brain, spinal cord, roots and peripheral nerves: Basic principles and procedures for routine clinical and research application. An updated report from an I.F.C.N. Committee. Clinical Neurophysiology. 2015;**126**(6):1071-1107

[12] Oliveri M et al. Magnetic stimulation study in patients with myotonic dystrophy. Electroencephalography and Clinical Neurophysiology. 1997;**105**(4):297-301

[13] Di Lazzaro V et al. Changes in motor cortex excitability in facioscapulohumeral muscular dystrophy. Neuromuscular Disorders. 2004;**14**(1):39-45

[14] Liepert J, Schoser BG, Weiller C. Motor excitability in myopathy. Clinical Neurophysiology. 2004;**115**(1):85-89

[15] Liepert J et al. Motor cortex excitability and fatigue in multiple sclerosis: A transcranial magnetic stimulation study. Multiple Sclerosis. 2005;**11**(3):316-321

[16] Maruyama A et al. Muscle fatigue decreases short-interval intracortical inhibition after exhaustive intermittent tasks. Clinical Neurophysiology. 2006;**117**(4):864-870

[17] Schwenkreis P et al. Central mechanisms during fatiguing muscle exercise in muscular dystrophy and fibromyalgia syndrome: A study with transcranial magnetic stimulation. Muscle & Nerve. 2011;**43**(4):479-484

[18] Boerio D et al. Central and peripheral components of exercise-related fatigability in myotonic dystrophy type 1. Acta Neurologica Scandinavica. 2012;**125**(1):38-46

[19] Lin KP et al. Fatigue in colchicine myopathy: A study of transcranial magnetic stimulation. Journal of the Chinese Medical Association. 2010;**73**(12):623-627

[20] Guidotti A et al. Isolation, characterization, and purification to homogeneity of an endogenous polypeptide with agonistic action on benzodiazepine receptors. Proceedings of the National Academy of Sciences of the United States of America. 1983;**80**(11):3531-3535

[21] Ono S et al. Neuropathological changes of the brain in myotonic dystrophy-some new observations. Journal of the Neurological Sciences. 1987;**81**(2-3):301-320

[22] Kassubek J et al. Quantification of brain atrophy in patients with myotonic dystrophy and proximal myotonic myopathy: A controlled 3-dimensional magnetic resonance imaging study. Neuroscience Letters. 2003;**348**(2):73-76

[23] Meola G et al. Executive dysfunction and avoidant personality trait in myotonic dystrophy type 1 (DM-1) and in proximal myotonic myopathy (PROMM/DM-2). Neuromuscular Disorders. 2003;**13**(10):813-821

[24] Liepert J et al. Central fatigue assessed by transcranial magnetic stimulation. Muscle & Nerve. 1996;**19**(11):1429-1434

[25] Di Lazzaro V et al. Direct demonstration of the effect of lorazepam on the excitability of the human motor cortex. Clinical Neurophysiology. 2000;**111**(5):794-799

[26] Di Lazzaro V et al. Origin of facilitation of motor-evoked potentials after paired magnetic stimulation: Direct recording of epidural activity in conscious humans. Journal of Neurophysiology. 2006;**96**(4):1765-1771

[27] Galaz-Vega R et al. Glutamate regulates dystrophin-71 levels in glia cells. Neurochemical Research. 2005;**30**(2):237-243

[28] Yoshihara Y et al. Abnormal kainic acid receptor density and reduced seizure susceptibility in dystrophin-deficient mdx mice. Neuroscience. 2003;**117**(2):391-395

[29] Rossi S et al. Safety, ethical considerations, and application guidelines for the use of transcranial magnetic stimulation in clinical practice and research. Clinical Neurophysiology. 2009;**120**(12):2008-2039

[30] Castel-Lacanal E et al. Induction of cortical plastic changes in wrist muscles by paired associative stimulation in the recovery phase of stroke patients. Neurorehabilitation and Neural Repair. 2009;**23**(4):366-372

[31] Fitzgerald PB, Fountain S, Daskalakis ZJ. A comprehensive review of the effects of rTMS on motor cortical excitability and inhibition. Clinical Neurophysiology. 2006;**117**(12):2584-2596

[32] Wagner T, Valero-Cabre A, Pascual-Leone A. Noninvasive human brain stimulation. Annual Review of Biomedical Engineering. 2007;**9**:527-565

[33] Hoogendam JM, Ramakers GM, Di Lazzaro V. Physiology of repetitive transcranial magnetic stimulation of the human brain. Brain Stimulation. 2010;**3**(2):95-118

Chapter 5

Ocular Pathology of Fukuyama Congenital Muscular Dystrophy

Tomoko Yamamoto, Yoichiro Kato and Noriyuki Shibata

Abstract

Fukuyama congenital muscular dystrophy (FCMD) is one of the congenital muscular dystrophies, showing central nervous system (CNS) and ocular lesions, in addition to muscular dystrophy. It is included in α-dystroglycanopathy, an entity of muscular dystrophies caused by reduced glycosylation of α-dystroglycan (α-DG). Studies of ocular lesions are not so many, compared with those of the muscle and CNS. Clinical ocular manifestations are myopia, strabismus, retinal detachment, and so on. Since the retina has a structure partly resembling the cerebral cortex, pathological findings similar to those found in the brain have been reported. The major observation considered to be involved in the pathogenesis of retinal lesions is abnormalities in the internal limiting membrane formed by Müller cells, which is corresponding to the glia limitans formed by astrocytes in the brain. Fukutin, responsible for FCMD, and α-DG are expressed in Müller cells. Moreover, fukutin may be involved in synaptic functions of retinal neurons through the glycosylation of α-DG. In this chapter, ocular lesions of fetal and child FCMD patients are presented, especially focusing on pathological findings of the retina, and functions of fukutin are discussed.

Keywords: eye, pathology, Fukuyama, muscular dystrophy, fukutin

1. Introduction

Fukuyama congenital muscular dystrophy (FCMD), described by Fukuyama et al., is an autosomal recessive disease, exclusively found in Japan [1, 2]. In addition to the muscular dystrophy, central nervous system (CNS) and eye anomalies are accompanied. Although there are mild to severe cases, patients are generally noticed as floppy infant, exhibit progressive muscular dystrophy and mental retardation, and die before 30 years [2]. The responsible gene is *fukutin* on chromosome 9q31 [3]. Among congenital muscular dystrophies, Walker Warburg syndrome (WWS) and muscle-eye-brain disease (MEB) show characteristics similar to FCMD [4, 5], although patients of FCMD show milder symptoms compared to those of WWS and MEB, in general [6]. Since responsible genes for WWS, MEB, and FCMD are implicated in the glycosylation of α-dystroglycan (α-DG), they are included in the entity of α-dystroglycanopathy [6].

At the sarcolemma of skeletal muscle, there is a complex composed of several proteins, including dystroglycans, sarcoglycans, and dystrophin. It is called the dystrophin-glycoprotein complex (DGC) that links extracellular matrix and intracellular proteins. The DGC is also observed in the CNS and in the eye.

The glycosylated area of α-DG existed outside the cell membrane works as a receptor for extracellular matrix proteins like laminin [6–8]. Thus, the glycosylation of α-DG is indispensable for formation of the basement membrane. To accomplish a fully glycosylated α-DG, several proteins, such as protein-O-mannosyltransferase 1/2 (POMT1/2) [9–11], O-linked mannose 1,2-N-acetylglucosaminyltransferase (POMGnT1) [12], fukutin [13], fukutin-related protein (FKRP) [14], and LARGE [15], are required. The recent study proves that fukutin transfers ribitol 5-phosphate to sugar chains of α-DG, which is necessary to make a functional α-DG [13].

Muscular dystrophies showing reduced glycosylation of α-DG due to malfunction of above proteins that add sugars on the glycosylation domain of α-DG are categorized to α-dystroglycanopathy, which include severe diseases like WWS, MEB, and FCMD to rather milder diseases like congenital muscular dystrophy 1C (MDC1C) [16], MDC1D [17], limb-girdle muscular dystrophy 2I (LGMD 2I) [16] LGMD2K, and LGMD2M [18]. In severe ones, CNS and eye anomalies are obvious. The CNS anomaly is represented by cortical dysplasia, generally called cobblestone lissencephaly [6, 7]. In FCMD, the cerebrum and cerebellum generally show an appearance of polymicrogyri [19–21]. In the surface of CNS, astrocytic endfeet form the glia limitans covered with the basement membrane, and both fukutin and α-DG are expressed in astrocytes [7, 22]. In the fetal FCMD brain, irregular disruptions of the glia limitans are observed. Neuronal tissues overmigrate from defects of glia limitans (**Figure 1**), which is considered to be the main cause of cobblestone lissencephaly [7, 8]. Hypoglycosylation of α-DG by malfunction of fukutin makes

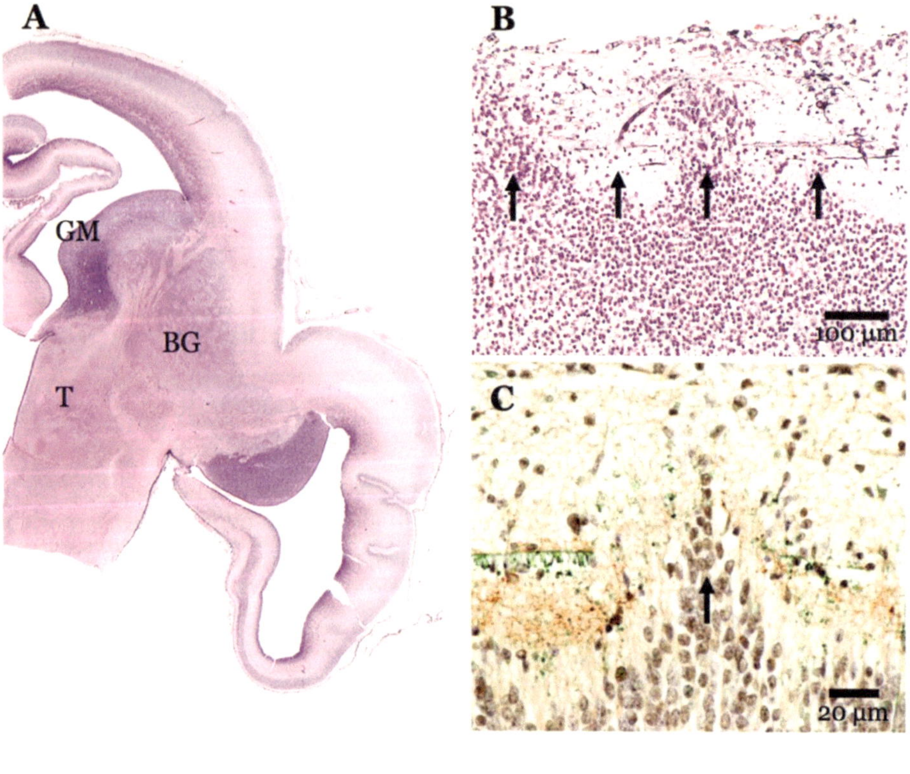

Figure 1.
Cerebral lesions of a FCMD fetus. The cerebral hemisphere almost retains fundamental structure (A). The glia limitans of the cerebral surface is irregularly disrupted, and neuronal tissues overmigrate through the disruptions (B, C; arrows). (B) Periodic acid-methenamine-silver (PAM) staining. (C) Photoshop-aided double immunostaining [25] of nestin (green) and synaptophysin (brown). BG: basal ganglia, GM: germinal matrix, T: thalamus.

the basement membrane fragile and this gives rise to partial defects in the glia limitans. Amounts of overmigrated neuronal tissues are various, depending on the size of defects [20, 23, 24].

Compared with the muscular and CNS lesions, studies about the ocular anomaly are rather scarce, but intriguing observations have been reported. Among the components of the eye, the retina has some characteristics common to the cerebral cortex. In this chapter, ocular lesions of FCMD are described, mainly focusing on retinal dysplasia and introducing resent studies on pathogenesis.

2. Normal development and structure of the eye

2.1 Normal development of the eye

Many genes are involved in the formation of ocular structure [26]. Morphologically, the initial eye structure becomes observable after 3 weeks of the gestation, as a pair of optic sulci at the rostral neural plate. By 4 weeks, the optic sulcus grows to form the optic vesicle, the proximal part of which develops to be the optic stalk, the future optic nerve, and the rest of which to be the optic cap. The distal part of the optic vesicle is closely adjacent to the surface ectoderm that develops to the lens after forming the lens vesicle by invagination. The lens vesicle is separated from the surface ectoderm at 6 and half weeks. The corneal epithelium begins to be formed from the surface ectoderm by 7 weeks. The choroid and the sclera develop from the periocular mesenchyme by 15 weeks.

The retina is differentiated from the optic cap. The inner layer of the optic cap becomes the neural retina, and the outer layer becomes the retinal pigmented epithelium. After retinal neurons are born, they move to their proper place, mimicking the development of CNS. However, the retina has its own mode for lamination [27]. In the retina, retinal ganglion cells and cone photoreceptors differentiate earlier, and then rod photoreceptors, bipolar cells, and Müller cells [26–28].

2.2 Normal structure of the eye

The eyeball can be divided into the anterior and posterior segments. The anterior segment includes the cornea, anterior and posterior chambers, iris, and lens. The posterior segment contains the vitreous, retina, choroid, sclera, and optic nerve (**Figure 2**).

Histologically, the normal retina consists of the inner and outer segments of photoreceptors, outer nuclear layer, outer plexiform layer, inner nuclear layer, inner plexiform layer, ganglion cell layer, and nerve fiber layer (**Figure 2**). Outer segments of the photoreceptor are loosely connected to retinal pigmented epithelia. Microvilli of the pigmented epithelium surround the outer segments of photoreceptors [29]. The outer nuclear layer contains nuclei of the photoreceptors, the rod and cone. Rods are extremely sensitive to light, while cones are involved in the color vision. In the outer plexiform layer, photoreceptors form synapses between bipolar cells: roughly, rods to rod bipolar cells and cones to cone bipolar cells. Rod bipolar cells depolarize (ON) to the increase of light intensity. On the other hand, cone bipolar cells either ON or hyperpolarize (OFF) [28]. The inner nuclear layer is mainly formed by bipolar cells. Cell bodies of amacrine cells, horizontal cells, and Müller cells are also contained. In the inner plexiform layer, synapses are formed between retinal ganglion cells and bipolar cells or amacrine cells. Synapses with ON-bipolar cells are seen in the inner lamina of the inner plexiform layer and those with OFF-bipolar cells in the outer lamina [28]. In the ganglion cell layer, single to several layers of retinal ganglion cells are observed. The nerve fiber layer consisted

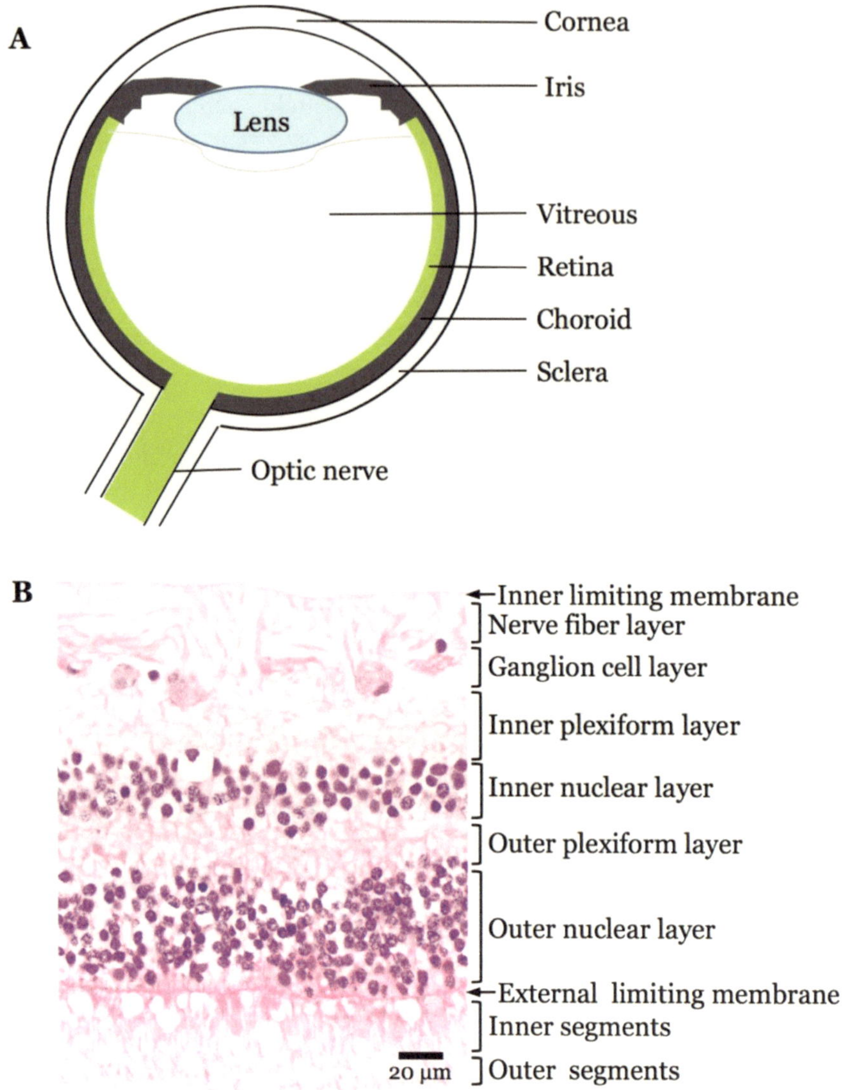

Figure 2.
(A) Schema of normal eye structure and (B) structure of normal retina.

of nerve fibers of retinal ganglion cells is situated beneath the inner limiting membrane that is formed at the inner surface of the retina by Müller cells. The external limiting membrane is formed by zonula adherens between Müller cells and inner segments of photoreceptor [29]. The basement membrane is abutted above the inner limiting membrane and beneath the basal surface of pigmented epithelium, attaching to the Bruch's membrane [29]. The basement membrane is also formed around capillaries.

3. Ocular lesions of FCMD

3.1 Clinical observations

In FCMD, both anterior and posterior components of the eye can be affected. Clinical symptoms include myopia, strabismus, and nystagmus [30–32]. Cataract, atrophy of the optic nerve, and retinal detachment are also known. Severe cases may show microphthalmia [31]. Electroretinogram (ERG) of FCMD patients may be normal, but abnormal findings may be seen in both dark-adapted and light-adapted ERGs [32]. Patients of WWS and MEB, severe forms of α-dystroglycanopathy, also exhibit abnormalities in anterior and posterior components. In WWS, varieties of lesions are described, such as cataract, microcornea, microphthalmia, retinal detachment, retinal dysplasia, and optic atrophy [4]. Glaucoma and buphthalmos also may be observed. Clinical ocular findings of MEB reported are myopia, nystagmus, optic atrophy, and retinal degeneration [33]. ERG is abnormal as well. Like the CNS, ocular anomalies of FCMD are less severe than those of WWS and MEB [30, 31].

3.2 Histological findings

Although histological examinations of the eye of fetal FCMD cases are not so many, findings similar to those of the cerebrum can be found [31]. The inner limiting membrane is irregularly disrupted and ganglion cells exist beyond the inner limiting membrane, while there are areas exhibiting no apparent light microscopical abnormalities (**Figure 3**). Like child cases, some fetal cases may show local folding and fusion of the retina [31].

In child FCMD cases, detachment, local folding, and fusion of the retina are observed (**Figure 4**). The inner limiting membrane is discontinuous. A persistent

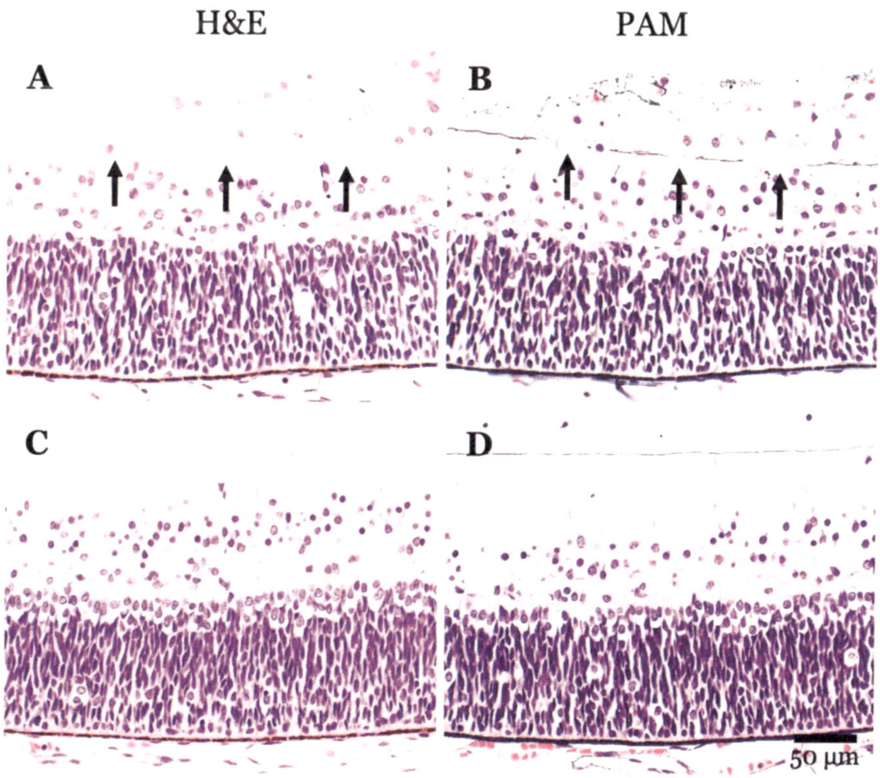

Figure 3.
Retinal findings in FCMD fetus. The internal limiting membrane, clearly depicted by PAM staining, is discontinuous in some part (A, B; arrows), while there are areas showing normal retinal appearance with continuous internal limiting membrane (C, D). Ectopic ganglion cells are observed beyond the inner limiting membrane.

hyperplastic primary vitreous body and a persistent hyaloid artery are also reported [31]. In severe cases, the layer of retina is markedly distorted with or without rosette formation. The outer and inner nuclear layers became thin in part. The layer of photoreceptor is also deranged with abnormal appearances of periodic acid-methenamine-silver (PAM)-positive structure (**Figure 4**). Reactive gliosis can be seen [31]. Severity of retinal dysplasia appears to be parallel to that of the CNS lesion [31].

3.3 Pathological consideration on retinal lesions of FCMD

In the CNS, fukutin and other related proteins are expressed in both glial cells and neurons [7, 34, 35]. Similarly, in the eye, fukutin is expressed in retinal neurons in addition to Müller cells [31, 36] (**Figure 5**).

Just above the inner limiting membrane formed by Müller cells abutted the basement membrane containing components of the DGC [37–39]. Like the CNS, abnormal basement membrane in the retinal surface may be involved in the pathogenesis of retinal dysplasia [31]. Focal fusion of the retina also may be caused by abnormal basement membrane. The glycosylation of α-DG is decreased in the inner limiting membrane of FCMD cases. Abnormalities of the basement membrane [40], decreased glycosylation of α-DG at the inner limiting membrane, and reactive gliosis [41] also have been reported in model mice of MEB. The study using α-dystroglycanopathy model mice and dystroglycan mutant mice suggest that DG is required for the maturation and maintenance of the inner limiting membrane, rather than its initial formation [42]. Retinal neurons can migrate properly under well-formed inner limiting membrane [42]. Although fukutin-null mice are lethal during pregnancy [43], the basic structure of retina and brain is relatively well kept in the early stage of the gestation of FCMD patients. Fukutin is considered to be essential for the embryogenesis. Severity of anomalies depends on a degree of functional loss of fukutin. On the brain of FCMD, lesions appear to be obvious after the second trimester. Strength of the surface structure may not catch up with the rapid increase of the volume of eye and brain. One of the interesting things is that the glycosylation of α-DG around the capillary is maintained. In POMGnT1 knock-out mice, the basement membrane of pigmented epithelium looks intact [40].

Müller cells have various roles to maintain retinal functions. One of the roles is to eliminate an excess of glutamate, a major transmitter in the retina, from the synaptic space. Glutamate is transported into Müller cells by glutamate transporter-1 (GLT-1) and metabolized to ornithine by ornithine aminotransferase (OAT) or to glutamine by glutamine synthase (GS). In FCMD patients, function of Müller cells seems to be decreased, because the expression of GLT-1, OAT, and GS is decreased [31].

In addition to the inner limiting membrane, the dystrophin-glycoprotein complex exists at presynaptic terminals of photoreceptor cells [41, 44]. As a ligand of α-DG, pikachurin is important for synaptic function between photoreceptor cells and bipolar cells [44]. In DG-knockout mice, pikachurin is markedly lost in both rod and cone photoreceptors with the loss of DG in these cells [44]. With the absence of DG, the retina becomes thin showing a decrease of photoreceptor cells, horizontal cells, and retinal ganglion cells in mice [42]. Decrease of ERG b-waves is observed in pikachurin-deficient mice and in dystroglycan-deficient mice [39]. Similar retinal lesions and abnormal ERGs are found in *fukutin*- [45], *POMGnT1*- [41], and *Pomt1*- [46] deficient mice, and *Large*^{myd} and *Large*^{vls} mice [47]. Hypoglycosylation of α-DG by hypofunction of fukutin and other proteins is considered to affect the function of retinal neurons as well as that of Müller cells.

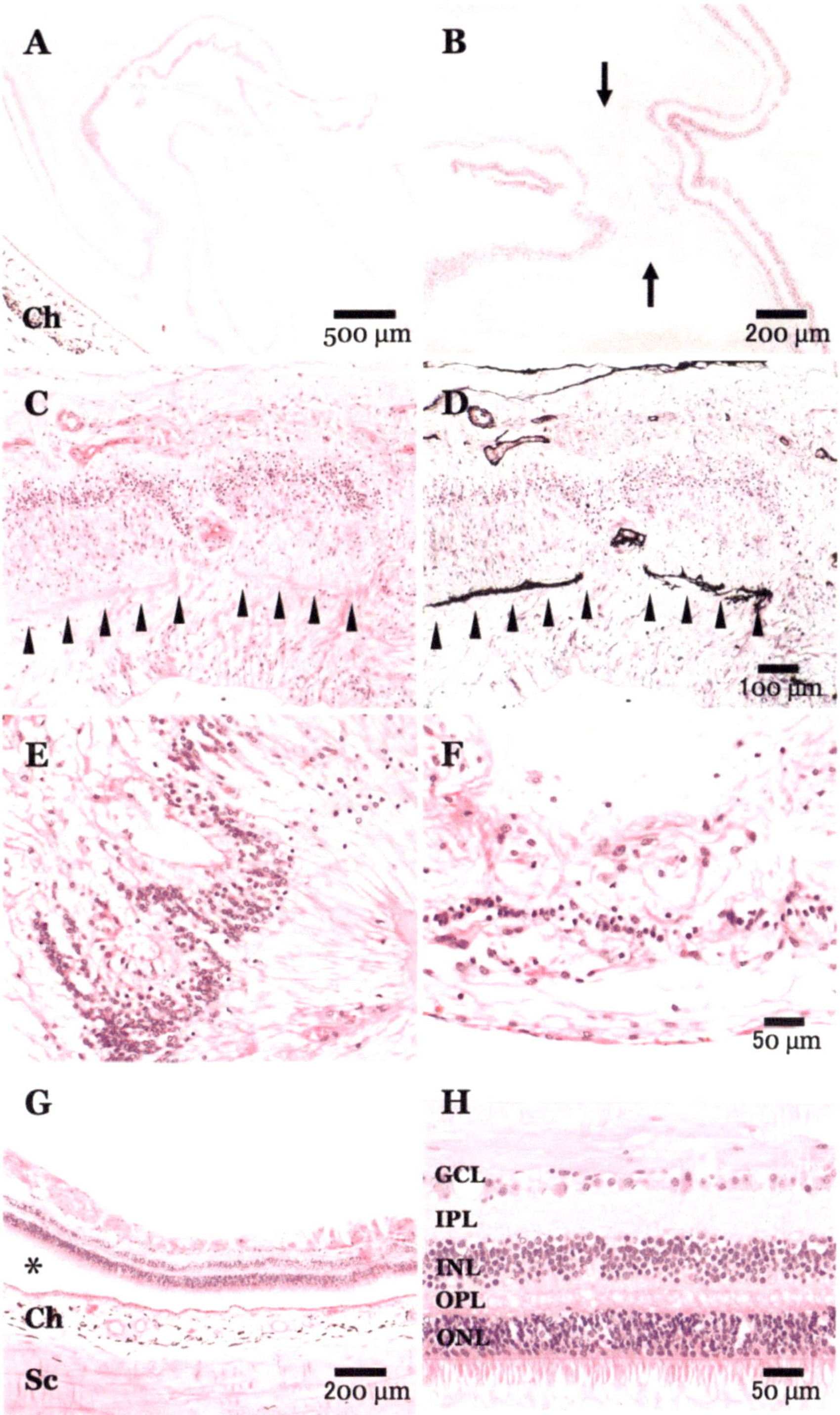

Figure 4.
Retinal findings in FCMD children. The retina is detached from the pigmented layer and abnormally folded (A, B), with focal surface fusion (arrows). In a severe case, retinal structure is abnormal with discontinuous PAM-positive structures, probably in the layer of photoreceptor cells. Normally, there is no such structure in this layer (C, D). Rosette structures are focally seen (E). The retina becomes thin with scarce retinal neurons (F). G and H show normal retina. The space indicated by the asterisk is an artifact during tissue preparation. Ch: choroid, Sc: sclera, GCL: ganglion cell layer, IPL: inner plexiform layer, INL: inner nuclear layer, OPL: outer plexiform layer, ONL: outer nuclear layer.

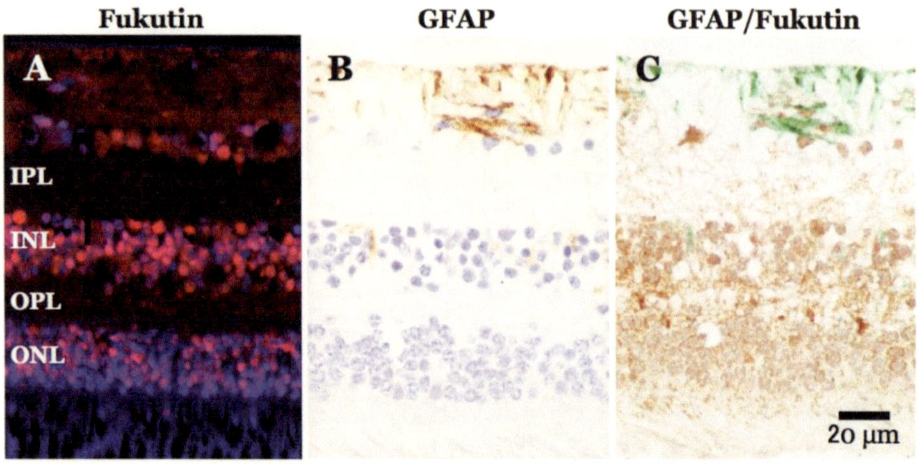

Figure 5.
Expression of fukutin in normal human retina. Fukutin is expressed in both retinal neurons and Müller cells (A–C). On fluorescent immunohistochemistry (A), fukutin is visualized in red (DAPI: blue). On Photoshop-aided double immunohistochemistry, green color indicates the elements positive for both fukutin and GFAP. IPL: inner plexiform layer, INL: inner nuclear layer, OPL: outer plexiform layer, ONL: outer nuclear layer.

Immunoreaction against antifukutin antibody is found in all the retinal layers, with stronger intensity in the inner segments of photoreceptors and in the outer plexiform layer [36]. In our immunostaining on formalin-fixed, paraffin-embedded human retina, all the layers are stained, but more intense in the outer and inner nuclear layer (**Figure 5**). This may due to the difference of tissue preparation like fixation. As for subcellular localization of fukutin, in retinal cells, it is mainly localized in the endoplasmic reticulum rather than the Golgi apparatus and in the nucleus *in vivo* [36]. Similar localization is observed in carcinoma cell lines [48]. These observations are contradict to the general consideration that fukutin is localized in the Golgi apparatus on cultured cells transfected with fukutin [3]. Further examinations are needed to explain the difference and clarify the localization of fukutin *in vivo*. If fukutin is truly localized in the endoplasmic reticulum and nucleus, this might suggest further unknown functions of fukutin, regardless of the relation to the glycosylation of α-DG.

4. Conclusions

Among severe forms of α-dystroglycanopathy like WWS, MEB, and FCMD, apparent CNS and ocular lesions are accompanied. Pathology of ocular lesions shares some characteristics common with that of CNS lesions. In this chapter, representative pathological findings of the eye of FCMD are presented, mainly focusing on the retinal dysplasia, and its pathogenesis is discussed with the review of literatures.

Acknowledgements

The authors wish to thank Ms. Noriko Sakayori, Mr. Fumiaki Muramatsu, Mr. Hideyuki Takeiri, Mr. Shuichi Iwasaki, and Mr. Mizuho Karita for their excellent technical assistance.

Conflict of interest

The authors declared that they have no conflict of interest.

Author details

Tomoko Yamamoto[1,2]*, Yoichiro Kato[2] and Noriyuki Shibata[1,2]

1 Department of Surgical Pathology, Tokyo Women's Medical University Hospital, Shinjuku-ku, Tokyo, Japan

2 Department of Pathology, Tokyo Women's Medical University, Shinjuku-ku, Tokyo, Japan

*Address all correspondence to: yamamoto.tomoko@twmu.ac.jp

References

[1] Fukuyama Y, Kawazura M, Haruna H. A peculiar form of congenital progressive muscular dystrophy. Paediatria Universitatis Tokyo. 1960;**4**: 5-8

[2] Osawa M, Sumida S, Suzuki N, Arai Y, Ikenaka H, Murasugi H, et al. Fukuyama type congenital progressive muscular dystrophy. In: Fukuyama Y, Osawa M, Saito K, editors. Congenital Muscular Dystrophies. Amsterdam: Elsevier; 1997. pp. 31-68

[3] Kobayashi K, Nakahori Y, Miyake M, Matsumura K, Kondo-Iida E, Nomura Y, et al. An ancient retro-transposal insertion causes Fukuyama-type congenital muscular dystrophy. Nature. 1998;**394**:388-392

[4] Vajsar J, Schachter H. Walker-Warburg syndrome. Orphanet Journal of Rare Diseases. 2006;**1**:29. DOI: 10.1186/1750-1172-1-29

[5] Taniguchi K, Kobayashi K, Saito K, Yamanouchi H, Ohnuma A, Hayashi YK, et al. Worldwide distribution and broader clinical spectrum of muscle-eye-brain disease. Human Molecular Genetics. 2003;**12**:527-534

[6] Martin PT. The dystroglycanopathies: The new disorders of O-linked glycosylation. Seminars in Pediatric Neurology. 2005; **12**:152-158

[7] Yamamoto T, Shibata N, Saito Y, Osawa M, Kobayashi M. Functions of fukutin, a gene responsible for Fukuyama type congenital muscular dystrophy, in neuromuscular system and other somatic organs. Central Nervous System Agents in Medicinal Chemistry. 2010;**10**:169-179

[8] Yamamoto T, Hiroi A, Kato Y, Shibata N, Osawa M, Kobayashi M. Possible divers roles of fukutin: More than basement membrane formation? In: Hedge M, Ankala A, editors. Muscular Dystrophy. Croatia: InTech; 2012. pp. 73-88

[9] Kim DS, Hayashi YK, Matsumoto H, Ogawa M, Noguchi S, Murakami N, et al. POMT1 mutation results in defective glycosylation and loss of laminin-binding activity in α- DG. Neurology. 2004;**62**:1009-1011

[10] Manya H, Chiba A, Yoshida A, Wang X, Chiba Y, Jigami Y, et al. Demonstration of mammalian protein *O*-mannosyltransferase activity: Coexpression of POMT1 and POMT2 required for enzymatic activity. Proceedings of the National Academy of Sciences of the United States of America. 2004;**101**:500-505

[11] van Reeuwijk J, Janssen M, van den Elzen C, Beltrán-Valero de Bernabé D, Sabatelli P, Merlini L, et al. *POMT2* mutations cause α-dystroglycan hypoglycosylation and Walker-Warburg syndrome. Journal of Medical Genetics. 2005;**42**:907-912

[12] Manya H, Sakai K, Kobayashi K, Taniguchi K, Kawakita M, Toda T, et al. Loss-of-function of an *N*-acetylglucosaminyltransferase, POMGnT1, in muscle-eye-brain disease. Biochemical and Biophysical Research Communications. 2003;**306**:93-97

[13] Kanagawa M, Kobayashi K, Tajiri M, Manya H, Kuga A, Yamaguchi Y, et al. Identification of a post-translational modification with ribitol-phosphate and its defect in muscular dystrophy. Cell Reports. 2016;**14**:2209-2223

[14] Brockington M, Blake DJ, Prandini P, Brown SC, Torelli S, Benson MA, et al. Mutations in the fukutin-related protein gene (*FKRP*) cause a form of

congenital muscular dystrophy with secondary lamininα2 deficiency and abnormal glycosylation of α-dystroglycan. American Journal of Human Genetics. 2001;**69**:1198-1209

[15] Peyrard M, Seroussi E, Sandberg-Nordqvist A-C, Xie Y-G, Han F-Y, Fransson I, et al. The human *LARGE* gene from 22q12.3-q13.1 is a new, distinct member of the glycosyltransferase gene family. Proceedings of the National Academy of Sciences of the United States of America. 1999;**96**:598-603

[16] Brockinton M, Yuva Y, Prandini P, Brown SC, Torelli S, Benson MA, et al. Mutations in the fukutin-related protein gene (*FKRP*) identify limb girdle muscular dystrophy 2I as a milder allelic variant of congenital muscular dystrophy MDC1C. Human Molecular Genetics. 2001;**10**:2851-2859

[17] Longman C, Brockington M, Torelli S, Jiménez-Mallebrera C, Kennedy C, Khalil N, et al. Mutations in the human *LARGE* gene cause MDC1D, a novel form of congenital muscular dystrophy with severe mental retardation and abnormal glycosylation of α-dystroglycan. Human Molecular Genetics. 2003;**12**:2853-2861

[18] Yis U, Uyanik G, Heck PB, Smitka M, Nobel H, Ebinger F, et al. *Fukutin* mutations in non-Japanese patients with congenital muscular dystrophy: Less severe mutations predominate in patients with a non-Walker-Warburg phenotype. Neuromuscular Disorders. 2011;**21**:20-30

[19] Kamoshita S, Konishi Y, Segawa M, Fukuyama Y. Congenital muscular dystrophy as a disease of the central nervous system. Archives of Neurology. 1976;**33**:513-516

[20] Takada K, Nakamura H, Tanaka J. Cortical dysplasia in congenital muscular dystrophy with central nervous system involvement (Fukuyama type). Journal of Neuropathology and Experimental Neurology. 1984;**43**:395-407

[21] Takada K, Nakamura H. Cerebellar micropolygyria in Fukuyama congenital muscular dystrophy: Observations in fetal and pediatric cases. Brain & Development. 1990;**12**:774-778

[22] Yamamoto T, Kawaguchi M, Sakayori N, Muramatsu F, Morikawa S, Kato Y, et al. Intracellular binding of fukutin and α-dystroglycan: Relation to glycosylation of α-dystroglycan. Neuroscience Research. 2006;**56**:391-399

[23] Takada K, Nakamura H, Suzumori K, Ishikawa T, Sugiyama N. Cortical dysplasia in a 23-week fetus with Fukuyama congenial muscular dystrophy (FCMD). Acta Neuropathologica. 1987;**74**:300-306

[24] Yamamoto T, Toyoda C, Kobayashi M, Kondo E, Saito K, Osawa M. Pial-glial barrier abnormalities in fetuses with Fukuyama congenital muscular dystrophy. Brain & Development. 1997;**19**:35-42

[25] Masuda A, Nishikawa T, Yamamoto T, Kobayashi M. Simple method for Photoshop-aided double immunohistochemistry—Usage of 'image stack' function. Histopathology. 2008;**53**:599-617

[26] Ohuchi H, Sato K, Habuta M, Fujita H, Bando T. Congenital eye anomalies: More mosaic than thought? Congenital Anomalies (Kyoto). 2018:1-18. DOI: 10.1111/cga.12304

[27] Amini R, Rocha-Martins R, Norden C. Neuronal migration and lamination in the vertebrate retina. Frontiers in Neuroscience. 2018;**11**:742. DOI: 10.3389/fnins.2017.00742

[28] Hoon M, Okawa H, Della Santina L, Wong ROL. Functional architecture of the retina: Development and disease. Progress in Retinal and Eye Research. 2014;**42**:44-84

[29] Green WR. Retina. In: Spencer WH, editor. Ophthalmic Pathology. An Atlas and Textbook. 3rd ed. Vol. 2. Philadelphia: WB Saunders; 1985. pp. 589-1291

[30] Yoshioka M, Kuroki S, Kondo T. Ocular manifestations in Fukuyama type congenital muscular dystrophy. Brain & Development. 1990;**12**:423-426

[31] Hino N, Kobayashi M, Shibata N, Yamamoto T, Saito K, Osawa M. Clinicopathological study on eyes from cases of Fukuyama type congenital muscular dystrophy. Brain & Development. 2001;**23**:97-107

[32] Kondo H, Saito K, Urano M, Sagara Y, Uchio E, Kondo M. A case of Fukuyama congenital muscular dystrophy associated with negative electroretinograms. Japanese Journal of Ophthalmology. 2010;**54**:622-637

[33] Fahnehjelm KT, Ygge J, Engman M-L, Mosskin M, Santavuori P, Malm G. A child with muscle-eye-brain disease. Acta Ophthalmologica Scandinavica. 2001;**79**:72-75

[34] Yamamoto T, Kato Y, Karita M, Kawaguchi M, Shibata N, Kobayashi M. Expression of genes related to muscular dystrophy with lissencephaly. Pediatric Neurology. 2004;**31**:183-190

[35] Moukhles H, Carbonetto S. Dystroglycan contributes to the formation of multiple dystrophin-like complexes in brain. Journal of Neurochemistry. 2001;**78**:824-834

[36] Haro C, Uribe ML, Quereda C, Cruces J, Martin-Nieto J. Expression in retinal neurons of fukutin and FKRP, the protein products of two dystroglycanopathy-causative genes. Molecular Vision. 2018;**24**:43-58

[37] Claudepierre T, Dalloz C, Mornet D, Matsumura K, Sahel J, Rendon A. Characterization of the intermolecular associations of the dystrophin-associated glycoprotein complex in retinal Müller glial cells. Journal of Cell Science. 2000;**113**:3409-3417

[38] Haenggi T, Fritschy J-M. Role of dystrophin and utrophin for assembly and function of the dystrophin glycoprotein complex in non-muscle tissue. Cellular and Molecular Life Sciences. 2006;**63**:1614-1631

[39] Satz JS, Philp AR, Nguyen H, Kusano H, Lee J, Turk R, et al. Visual impairment in the absence of dystroglycan. The Journal of Neuroscience. 2009;**29**:13136-13146

[40] Hu H, Candiello J, Zhang P, Ball SL, Cameron DA, Halfter W. Retinal ectopias and mechanically weakened basement membrane in a mouse model of muscle-eye-brain (MEB) disease congenital muscular dystrophy. Molecular Vision. 2010;**16**:1415-1428

[41] Takahashi H, Kanesaki H, Igarashi T, Kameya S, Yamaki K, Mizota A, et al. Reactive gliosis of astrocytes and Müller glial cells in retina of POMGnT1-deficient mice. Molecular and Cellular Neurosciences. 2011;**47**:119-130

[42] Clements R, Turk R, Campbell KP, Wright KM. Dystroglycan maintains inner limiting membrane integrity to coordinate retinal development. The Journal of Neuroscience. 2017;**37**: 8559-8574

[43] Kurahashi H, Taniguchi M, Meno C, Taniguchi Y, Takeda S, Horie M, et al. Basement membrane fragility underlies embryonic lethality in *fukutin*-null mice. Neurobiology of Disease. 2005;**19**: 208-217

[44] Omori Y, Araki F, Chaya T, Kajimura N, Irie S, Terada K, et al. Presynaptic dystroglycan–pikachurin complex regulates the proper synaptic connection between retinal photoreceptor and bipolar cells. The Journal of Neuroscience. 2012;**32**: 6126-6137

[45] Takeda S, Kondo M, Sasaki J, Hirahashi H, Kano H, Arai K, et al. Fukutin is required for maintenance of muscle integrity, cortical histogenesis and normal eye development. Human Molecular Genetics. 2003;**12**:1449-1459

[46] Rubio-Fernández M, Uribe ML, Vicente-Tejedor J, Germain F, Susín-Lara C, Quereda C, et al. Impairment of photoreceptor ribbon synapses in a novel *Pomt1* conditional knockout mouse model of dystroglycanopathy. Scientific Reports. 2018;**8**:8543. DOI: 10.1038/s41598-018-26855-x

[47] Lee Y, Kameya S, Cox GA, Hsu J, Hicks W, Maddatu TP, et al. Ocular abnormalities in *Large*^{myd} and *Large*^{vls} mice, spontaneous models for muscle, eye, and brain diseases. Molecular and Cellular Neurosciences. 2005;**30**:160-172

[48] Yamamoto T, Kato Y, Shibata N, Sawada T, Osawa M, Kobayashi M. A role of fukutin, a gene responsible for Fukuyama type congenital muscular dystrophy, in cancer cells: A possible role to suppress cell proliferation. International Journal of Experimental Pathology. 2008;**89**:332-341

Section 4

Therapeutic Approaches for Muscular Dystrophy

Chapter 6

Physical Exercise as a Tool to Delay the Development Process of Duchenne Muscular Dystrophy

Samuel Alexandre Almeida Honório, Marco Batista, Jorge Santos, João Petrica, Helena Mesquita, João Serrano, Jaime Ribeiro and Júlio Martins

Abstract

Several authors reported that the absence of normal physical activity promotes a faster functional loss of several organs and systems, such as the cardiorespiratory system. It is known that scheduling physical activities and regular exercise for DMD patients, when performed based on a thorough functional evaluation, is fundamental for maintaining the quality of life of these children, as well as other associated resources that should be used, whenever possible. Exercise can help DMD patients to maintain and improve muscular strength for performing activities of daily living (ADL) such as stair climbing, slow the rate of increased weakness or contracture development that can prolong ambulation, maintain enough respiratory capacity and strengthened postural muscles, which can slow the onset of scoliosis. There is a need to pass throughout the message to professionals, staff and families who are in this context or who have children with developmental disabilities that exercise and physical activity are an essential factor for maintaining health and well-being throughout the lifespan. That's what we wish and hope with this chapter.

Keywords: exercise, Duchenne muscular dystrophy, physical activity, movement, life quality

1. Introduction

It is known that there are a growing number of parents looking for ways to improve their children's quality of life because of Duchenne muscular dystrophy's consequences.

As a tool, exercise in aquatic environment allows children to achieve skills that can be difficult on the ground. With this in mind, a literature review was carried out to systematize the pediatric sequelae that can be treated with the benefits of physical activity in Duchenne muscular dystrophy [1–4].

Aquatic activity has been a way of stimulating the development of children and expanding the experiences of healthy, disabled or at-risk children [5]. The premature child and those who are at high risk of neurological injury or developmental delay may already have experienced hydrotherapy as an intensive care intervention. Very young babies participate together with their parents in aquatic programs. Within the exercise techniques, it is hydrotherapy that enables the accomplishment of activities of greater degree of difficulty, providing patients with psychological benefits. If compared to techniques performed on the ground, hydrotherapy due to the physical principles of water facilitates and improves balance, coordination and posture and gives the patient the feeling of safety. For the child the feeling of safety is found in the arms of the parents and in the contact with the body. This was experienced in the sensation of water environment, before birth, and is now again found in the heat of the water.

2. Exercise for Duchenne muscular dystrophy

Hydrotherapy is a classic form of treatment, used with large varieties of functions [6]. The physical properties of heated water promote a facilitating movement and relief of pain, as well as allowing group work and making therapy pleasant, especially for children, who are often unable to perform certain activities in another environment, if not the aquatic. In this study, the effects of immersion in warm water in children with Duchenne muscular dystrophy were measured using HR, O2 saturation, maximal inspiratory pressure (MIP), maximal expiratory pressure (MEP) and oral temperature (OT) measurements. A total of 20 children with Duchenne muscular dystrophy, male, aged 8 to 15 years, participated in this study.

Regarding the heart rate, a mean decrease of 7.3 bpm was observed between the initial immersion period and the pre-immersion period; between the final immersion period and the beginning of the immersion, there was an average increase of 7 bpm and observed a mean decrease of 0.3 bpm between the pre-immersion and final immersion periods. The oral temperature showed an increase of 0.1° C, during the initial immersion period; in relation to the pre-immersion period, this increase is probably associated with the immersion in warm water added to the physical activity, a decrease of 0.1°C between the final immersion period and the initial immersion period.

The O2 saturation showed a decrease in the values obtained after immersion, where there was a decrease of 2.7 between the initial immersion period and the pre-immersion; a 0.9% increase occurred between the initial and final immersion periods and one increase of 1.8% between the values of the final and pre-immersion periods, which were also considered measures of normal physiological adjustments to physical activities.

At the maximum inspiratory pressure, there was a mean decrease of 8 cm of water between the initial period of immersion and the pre-immersion; this change was considered clinically significant; between the periods of immersion, an average increase of 3.8 cm of water was observed of maximal inspiratory pressure.

At the maximum expiratory pressure in relation to the values obtained between the pre-immersion and initial immersion periods, we obtained an increase of 7.4 cm of water, and subsequently between the immersion and thin periods, there was a drop of 6.8 cm of water. This study showed that hydrotherapy is a therapeutic resource that does not represent an overload for children with Duchenne muscular dystrophy. Another study [7] was aimed to verify the benefits of hydrotherapy in improving gait and balance in patients with mild spastic diplegic type of muscular dystrophy, using a proposed protocol. The objective of this study was to analyze the changes in movements in the lower limbs during gait through a treatment protocol using aquatic rehabilitation, to help the child to achieve better gait independence, for which a case study was used, selecting a male child with gait changes.

The protocol was based on relaxation for 5 minutes: muscle stretching of ankle flexors, ankle dorsiflexors, hip adductors, hip and trunk flexors; passive ankle, plantar and dorsiflexion and circular movements; pelvic girdle dissociation; muscle strengthening of hip and knee extensors and abductors and bicycle and gait training associated with balance training using a 1-pound ankle support and water turbulence. The patient was submitted to the protocol twice a week, lasting 50 minutes each session, totaling seven sessions.

In the initial evaluation, it was observed that the patient, in his functional activities, acquired all the positions without aid except the standing position and the gait. In the evaluation of the gait after the treatment compared to the initial evaluation, it was verified that there were no changes in gait phases. However, when analyzing the patient in the sagittal plane, it is emphasized that the patient used the support of one hand; there was a moment when he wandered without support, evidencing an improvement in the balance. In this study it can be concluded that the application of the proposed protocol in the hydrotherapeutic rehabilitation of the gait was considered efficient due to the good results obtained and proven in the reevaluation as an increase in balance and gait control.

Other authors [8] evaluated individuals with muscle tone disorders, posture and voluntary movement. These disorders are characterized by the lack of control over the movements, by adaptive modifications of the muscular length, resulting in some cases in bone deformities. Neuromotor involvement of this disease may involve distinct parts of the body, resulting in specific topographical classifications (quadriplegia, hemiplegia and diplegia). A child with DMD with diagnosis of hemiplegia, male, 8 months of age, participated in this study. In the therapy performed, a swimming pool with water between 30 and 32°C degrees was used, twice a week with a duration of 30 minutes in the period of August to December of 2004, totaling 40 sessions.

The hydrotherapy sessions consisted of joint mobilizations, stretches, active exercises, Halliwick concept and Bad Ragaz ring method and neuro-evolutionary Bobath treatment adapted in the water with a duration of 30 minutes.

After the hydrotherapy treatment, the child achieved in the area of personal care the following acquisitions: variability of food textures and use of spoon in food, holding an object against gravity and gains in personal hygiene by acquiring partial brushing of teeth and hair and participation in bathing and dressing. It was noted in the area of mobility the condition of sitting in vehicles and moving within it. He was also able to perform transfers from posture to sitting and transfer from the ground to the bed and vice versa, independence in locomotion in internal and external environments, gain of the distance walked. In the social function area, the child acquired comprehension of word meanings and increased vocabulary, comprising complex sentences, aptly naming objects, concomitantly making use of appropriate gestures and problem solving, resulting in greater interaction with children of his or her age. The analysis of this study can be concluded that the application of hydrotherapy in hemiplegic patients provided a sensorimotor improvement in existing functional skills, as well as in the acquisition of others. Thus, the child was better adapted to its development.

According with this line of investigation, another author [9] sought to correlate fat mass and muscle strength, maximum respiratory pressures and respiratory function in individuals with DMD. We selected 68 subjects with DMD. Muscle strength was assessed through manual tests, maximal respiratory pressures through a vacuum gauge and the Vignos test collected by observation. The fat mass was evaluated by bioimpedance, and BMI was also evaluated. Descriptive statistical analysis and regression model construction were performed. A descriptive analysis of the data was performed, and the subjects were divided by quartiles of age. There was a significant correlation between the dependent values, fat percentage and age. Based on this study, it was concluded that there is a correlation between the percentage of fat and muscle strength, respiratory pressures and respiratory function in subjects with DMD.

Another research [10] studied the correlation between fat mass and age in Duchenne muscular dystrophy. Were selected 68 individuals with ages between 5 and 20 years, with molecular diagnosis of DMD. All were submitted to weight and height measurements and to the body composition analysis test with the use of bioimpedance, in the morning, all on the same day. The results were analyzed by grouping the individuals into quartiles of age and showed a body mass index (BMI) of 21 ± 8 kg/m^2. Thus, it was observed that, with the age and degree of sedentarism imposed by the disease, there was an accumulation of body fat and loss of lean mass. They understand that, in fact, more studies are needed related to the nutritional characteristics of these individuals, in order to better clarify the effects of disease and feeding on the percentage gain and fat mass.

An investigation [11] was conducted to evaluate respiratory muscle strength and peak flow in patients with Duchenne muscular dystrophy undergoing noninvasive ventilation and hydrotherapy. Six volunteers of male gender, aged between 13 and 19, were divided into two groups: control (treated with hydrotherapy) and experimental (treated with hydrotherapy associated with NIV), which were evaluated before and after the 10th and 20th sessions. The results showed a significant difference ($p < 0.05$) when we compared MEP between the control and experimental groups after the 10th ($p = 0.025$) and the 20th ($p = 0.005$) sessions. The study demonstrated that NIV was able to influence an increase in life expectancy, according to the patients' own reports, and that hydrotherapy was a favorable therapy in the improvement of the expiratory musculature in patients with DMD. For this purpose, physical activities were carried out once a week in a pool, with a duration of 30 minutes. The main objective was to maintain and stimulate the patient's respiratory function, which was exercised without the use of a life-saving vest or other type of fluid. The pool height was 110 cm in the shallow part and 115 cm in the deepest part. The water was kept warm at 34°C. The activities were carried out with a group of three children besides the teacher. For warm-up exercises, for 10 minutes, involving movements of the body segments, the following activities were carried out to collect rings at the bottom of the pool, to pass under and over flutuators organized in sequence, to enter and exit the flutuators, to blow balls and fish of floating material and to sink balls. For each of these activities, it was requested to perform inspiration out of the water and exhale with the whole body inside the water. In this way the water exerted pressure against the rib cage, and the inspiration occurred against the resistance. At the end, in the period of 3 to 4 minutes, relaxation was carried out with the student floating in the pool. Six measurements were performed, once a month. The first occurred on July 8, 2001, and the last on December 5, 2001. The values were obtained for respiratory rate per minute and vital capacity. No changes were observed in the value of vital capacity between the first and last evaluations, remaining in 800 cm3. Regarding respiratory rate, a decrease from 29 to 26 cycles per minute was observed. It was observed that there was an increase in the thoracic perimeter in normal inspiration and deep inspiration over the 6 months. There was an increase of 1.5 cm in the thoracic perimeter in the normal inspiration and the values obtained in the thoracic perimeter evaluations. According to the author [12] who studies the muscular attrition associated to DMD starts at the beginning of the second childhood and respiratory muscle weakness leads to a series of events that culminate in respiratory complications that worsen considerably at around 10 to 19 years of age. The respiratory complications presented by DMD patients are due, in part, to muscle weakness and thoracic cavity changes caused by scoliosis that affects the patient with disease progression [13].

In another study [14] authors sought to determine the effects of pool physical exercises on the pulmonary function of the person with Duchenne muscular dystrophy. Physiotherapeutic treatment has proven to be important not only in-patient rehabilitation but also in the prevention of imperative changes in this pathology and in teaching to the family, because better results are expected if the parents cooperate.

Examinations of neurodevelopmental status, locomotor system, functional capacity and respiratory system are therefore important. Only then can the main problems be identified, to collect the necessary information and then structure the treatment objectives, which vary according to each specific case. Thus, several protocols have been introduced in order to document the evolution of neuromuscular diseases. Timed functional tests and specific rating scales were designed to document decreased functional capacity. Developed in 1963, the "Vignos Scale for the Classification of Duchenne Muscular Dystrophy Cases" was elaborated [15] which determines the functional degrees of limbs. Repeated studies were developed to determine the reliability of the functional tests, including the Vignos scale, which demonstrated a high degree of reliability. Manual muscle testing (MMT) and its quantitative muscle testing (QMT) were also applied in order to determine its usefulness and reliability to document the evolution of functional decay.

Quantitative muscle testing (QMT) includes determination of isometric strength and is the most direct method to examine the contractile activity of a particular muscle group. It has the advantage of muscle length, joint angle and speed of being kept constant. This test requires the application of special equipment such as an ergometer.

Tests that examine respiratory function, including forced vital capacity (FVC) and forced expiratory volume (FEV) per second, determined with the help of the vitalograph, provide information about the strength of the respiratory muscles. It may be equally interesting to determine the endurance capacity of the respiratory muscles. For professional evaluation of the examination plan to be used, the child's age, ability to follow instructions, availability of equipment, place of examination (clinic, residence, school), available time and (for research purposes or to serve as a basis for treatment) need to previously assessed.

Currently, some specialized sites have a specific record of evaluation of these neuromuscular pathologies, the "MRC grading muscle strength". This sheet assesses the strength of different muscle groups of the upper and lower limbs and head and trunk but also refers to joint limitations caused by contractures as well as motor skills.

Although these assessments are quite comprehensive and complex, they should be repeated regularly for a correct planning of the treatment, according to the current needs of the individual in question. These needs vary according to the stage of the patient, and their treatment must be adapted.

3. Hydrotherapy on Duchenne muscular dystrophy cases: a summary proposal for intervention

Hydrotherapy with temperatures above 30°C will have a beneficial effect on circulation and will improve the elasticity of connective tissue. Particular attention should be paid to the excessive weariness of the child, which very hot water can cause, since fatigue is harmful.

Muscle strengthening techniques are not indicated, as it is reported that they worsen muscle degradation. It is extremely important to prevent contractures and deformities. In this way the exercises should be performed in the most affected regions of the body such as:

Tibiotarsus and feet—the use of instrumental positions with wedges and in vertical or inclined plane, thus using body weight. When the child is seated, the feet should be supported in a neutral position of the tibiotarsus and without abduction of the hips. The purpose of this care is to prolong verticalization, the use of footwear and the absence of pain in the region.

Knees—usually only needed after loss of gait to prevent flexion by retraction of the hamstrings, allowing prolongation of the verticalization and adoption of a more comfortable sleeping position, manual stretching posture and posture with weights in a sitting position, with the basin in retroversion and the lower limbs aligned.

Ankle—in small children it is possible to do the manual stretching in the ventral decubitus, with the knee in 90° bending. In greater angles the instrumental stance is necessary and in passive mobilization. The use of the ventral decubitus should be recommended whenever possible for sleeping, watching television, reading, etc.

Spine—changes occur after loss of gait. The use of orthoses, which can be the shaped vest, is of controversial interest. During the reducible phase, the manual positions of flank opening in the concavity and the passive traction are used.

Shoulders—tardily after loss of gait, make manual stretches of upper trapezius.

Elbows—also after loss of gait. The aim is not to totally avoid bending but to stagnate the angle at which there is the best lever arm for the weakened flexor muscles. Already the supination deficit must be combated, with mobilization and manual postures.

It is also not a goal to completely combat the retraction of the flexors and extensors of the wrist, since from a certain point the tenodesis grasp (passive hand grasp and release induced by wrist extension or flexion) may be the only one possible.

Hydrotherapy is also important in terms of respiratory function, as it depends on the efficacy of respiratory muscles, as well as the degree of bronchial obstruction, once is known the hydrostatic pressure factor on the rib cage. Because of the initial deficit of forced expiration and cough efficacy, maintenance of bronchial clearance is particularly important from early stages. Subsequently, the ability to inhale deeply is lost.

This is particularly important if we note that in the lung development process, the number of pulmonary alveoli stabilizes at about 8 years of age and then increases in size to adult size. If deep inspirations are not performed, which are important for this increase, the alveolar growth is not so great, being a factor of aggravation of the restrictive disease and of the thoracic deformity.

Hydrotherapy should be done regularly as it improves the technique of bronchial clearance and acceleration of the expiratory flow, causing an active (possible while walking) or passive expiration, which causes the secretions to be released up to the coughing zone. Previously, the secretions must be humidified with air or with flutuators. Percussions are often traumatic and vibrations alone are not productive.

The amplitude maintenance techniques are initially activated and then performed using ventilatory assist devices. When vital capacity equals tidal volume, measures may be taken to establish permanent ventilation.

Until a few years ago, physical treatment of DMD was aimed at preserving and stimulating mobility and motility (as far as possible) through "corrective gymnastics, swimming, prophylaxis of contractures, combating inactivity and unnecessary bed rest" [5] which consisted of nondrug treatment. However, physical therapy is much more than "corrective gymnastics", "swimming" and "combating inactivity". Physical therapy traces treatment with goal-based conduits.

The goal of physical therapy is to enable the child to gain control over his or her possible movements, balance and general coordination, delay weakness of the pelvic girdle and scapular muscles, correct postural alignment (standing, sitting, lying down or during movements), balancing muscle work, avoid fatigue, develop the contractile force of respiratory muscles and control breathing through the correct use of the diaphragm and prevent early muscle shortening.

To achieve these goals, a playful treatment is proposed to indulge playfulness of these patients, as they are still children and become bored easily. Physiotherapeutic procedures should be adapted to the age range of the child and are mainly aimed at delaying clinical evolution and preventing secondary complications (contractures and deformities). In some cases, corrective surgeries and orthotics assist in the treatment.

Free active and isometric exercises are proposed. Playing a wooden doll, because the movements are monoarticular, requires the contraction of a muscle or a reduced group of muscles; on quadruped or weight-bearing position, as it strengthens the scapular and pelvic girdle. During the execution of these exercises, one must seek to evaluate the range of motion (ROM) and muscle strength, request isometric contractions during movements and make use of weight segments as resistance for the muscle group exercised.

The specific respiratory exercises include motivation, such as "flower smelling" and "blow the candle", provided that in dorsal decubitus at 45° of inclination, neither the inspiratory reserve volume nor the expiratory reserve volume (VRE), without using the accessory muscles, nor do resistance to expiration. Taking this into account, it's important to highlight that the effects of inspiratory resistance training on respiratory muscle function were investigated. The authors [11] evaluated 11 patients with DMD and facioscapulohumeral muscular dystrophy, after respiratory training, which consisted of 2 sessions of 15 min per day at home for 6 weeks; there was a significant increase in respiratory muscle endurance, positively correlated with vital capacity ($r = 0.84$, $p < 0.05$) and maximal inspiratory pressure ($r = 0.76$, $p < 0.05$). According to the authors, the improvement of respiratory muscle function may delay the installation of respiratory complications in these patients. In another study on respiratory muscle training with patients with DMD and spinal muscular atrophy, it was found that gains in expiratory muscle strength were rapidly lost with the end of treatment. However, the perception of respiratory effort remained for a longer period, which could be associated with a reduction of respiratory symptoms. In a 6-month study of specific inspiratory muscle training in DMD patients in the advanced stages, the authors realized that, even after 6 months of termination of the training protocol, the respiratory benefits remained for a long period of time.

The activities in the therapeutic balls favor the alignment and flexibility of the spine, stimulate the mechanoreceptors and articular proprioceptors and improve tone and muscle strength, coordination and balance.

The use of hydrotherapy, using methods adapted from Halliwick and Bad Ragaz, is a complementary feature to ground kinesiotherapy, in order to improve muscle strength, respiratory capacity and joint amplitudes and avoid muscular shortening.

The causes of orthopedic contractures in neurological patients are immobilization, muscle weakness and spasticity. The literature describes techniques of treatment of contractures passive stretching, continuous passive mobilization, splinting, electrical stimulation, botulinum toxin injections and tenotomies. There is no consensus on the best way to use the techniques of treatment of contractures, whether combined or isolated in series. Stretching of the sural triceps, ilium-psoas and tibialis-ischemia should be stimulated in the early stages. Short, ankle-foot orthosis (AFO) or long knee-ankle-foot orthosis (KOFO) should be worn at night to prevent muscle shortening. For postural alignment, instruct the child not to stay too long in the same position and give the child the highest body awareness possible. Parents should be instructed and trained to continue home treatment and to encourage their children to engage in age-oriented recreational activities that provide balance, strength and coarse motor coordination. One study [16] followed 204 children with DMD for a period of 8.9 years on average at a research center in the United States. It was able to monitor the effects of physical therapy and orthopedic treatment on lower limb contractures (LLC) and the duration of walking ability. MMI contractures were better controlled when patients performed a combination

	Type	Frequency	Intensity	Duration
Flexibility	Passive/active	Daily	Low	3x (10–30 seg)
Resistance exercises	Short walking Hydrotherapy	Variable 1–6 per week	Low	Variable 1–20 minutes
Muscular strength	Isokinetic	Variable 1–5 per week	Low	Variable 1–3 series 5–15 repetitions

Table 1.
General exercises guidelines for patients with DMD [18].

of daily passive stretches, stood and walked for some periods of the day, had a tenotomy of the calcaneus tendon, transferred posterior tibial tendon and applied KAFO-type orthoses. After 2 years of the use of bracing, the calcaneus contractures were identical in those patients who performed and who did not perform surgeries. Near the fourth-year post-bracing, however, patients who did not undergo surgery had more severe contractures. Five to 7 years after the operation and the use of bracing, the management of contractures was still good, especially in those patients who performed posterior tibial tendon transfer.

Knee contractions were controlled 5 to 7 years after the placement of bracing, with or without surgery. Patients who used bracing were able to walk for an average of 13.6 years, and even after they lost the ability to walk with bracing, the use of orthoses allowed these patients to remain in orthostasis for an additional 2 years. Another study [17] also reinforces the prolongation of gait and orthostasis with the aid of KAFO-type orthoses, but there is no clarification as to whether it is possible to prolong gait functionally.

These procedures are just suggestions. It is up to the technician to choose the most suitable resources available to his/her patients. It is important to note that fatigue and myalgia on the day after the physical therapy session indicate that there was an excess in the number of exercises and their repetitions and that the intensity should be decreased and have more time to rest. Therefore, the main objective to be achieved is to improve the quality of life and the functionality of these children. The quality of life of an adult can be improved by increasing their independence. For the child, the improvement of their quality of life implies the action of playing, however, in a functional way.

In the late stages of the life of the DMD patient, the goal is to comfort the patient: treat pain and dyspnoea, provide palliative care, meet the psychosocial and spiritual needs of the patient and family and respect the patient's and family's choices in what examination and treatment (**Table 1**).

4. Conclusions

A literary survey can be observed that the treatment in pediatrics with the use of hydrotherapy is quite effective in the pathologies that were mentioned for the accomplishment of this work. It can be concluded that the treatment of children in aquatic environment has a great value, due to its positive effects.

Neurofunctional intervention has much to do with DMD and DMB, as patients with these conditions cannot be seen only due to their limitations caused by neurological diseases, which need not only motor care. They need to be seen as people who need interdisciplinary action, since complications occur in the orthopedic and cardiorespiratory fields (not counting other needs, such as psychological and nutritional monitoring).

Special tests, which allow for more precise monitoring of the evolution of the disease, and tools that evaluate the quality of life should be used not only in academic circles. However, they exist to facilitate the recording of information, for later publications in professional scope.

As the natural evolution of these pathologies is already known, it justified the increasingly early performance of the physiotherapist. We also have the task of guiding the caregivers of these children (parents, teachers and family) and referring to the occupational therapist, so that the necessary adaptations are made in the homes, schools and bathrooms. In addition, play adaptations and physical activity can improve the social life of these children.

Acknowledgements

This work is supported by national funding through Portuguese Foundation for Science and Technology, IP., DTP/04045/2019 and UID/CED/00194/2019.

Conflict of interest

The authors declare no conflict of interests.

Author details

Samuel Alexandre Almeida Honório[1*], Marco Batista[1], Jorge Santos[1], João Petrica[1], Helena Mesquita[2], João Serrano[1], Jaime Ribeiro[3,4] and Júlio Martins[5]

1 Polytechnic Institute of Castelo Branco, SHERU (Sport, Health and Exercise Research Unit), Castelo Branco, Portugal

2 Polytechnic Institute of Castelo Branco, Interdisciplinary Centre of Social Sciences (CICS.NOVA)/SHERU (Sport, Health and Exercise Research Unit), Castelo Branco, Portugal

3 School of Health Sciences and Centre for Innovative Care and Health Technology (CiTechCare), Polytechnic of Leiria, Portugal

4 Research Centre on Didactics and Technology in the Education of Trainers (CIDTFF), University of Aveiro, Portugal

5 University of Beira Interior, CIDESD, Covilhã, Portugal

*Address all correspondence to: samuelhonorio@hotmail.com

References

[1] Cunha A. Avaliação da funcionalidade de uma criança com hemiplegia espástica à direita com tratamento hidroterapêutico, estudo de caso [thesis]. Brasil: Instituto de Pesquisa e Desenvolvimento da Universidade do Vale do Paraíba; 2002

[2] Caromano F, Lilia K, Passarella C. Efeitos fisiológicos de sessão de hidroterapia em crianças portadoras de distrofia muscular de duchenne. Revista Fisioterapia. 1998;**1**:49-55

[3] Honório S. Estudo Longitudinal da Influência da Actividade Física, o IMC e a Percentagem de Massa Gorda na Correlação entre a Escala Motora Funcional EK em Indivíduos com Distrofia Muscular de Duchenne [Tese de Doutoramento]. Covilhã: Universidade da Beira Interior; 2012

[4] Ovando A. A hidroterapia como forma de tratamento para Distrofia muscular de Duchenne: Relato de caso. Revista Efdeportes. 2008;**4**:23-35

[5] Cardoso A, Rodolfo L, Andréa C, Bruna F, Daiane N, Regiane A. hidroterapia na reabilitação do equilíbrio na marcha do portador de paralisia cerebral diplégica espástica leve. XI Encontro Latino Americano de Iniciação Cientifica e VII Encontro Latino Americano de Pós-Graduação; 12 a 15 de Maio de 2002; Universidade do Vale do Paraná, Brasil

[6] Okama L. Avaliação funcional e postural nas distrofias musculares de Duchenne e Becker. ConScientiae Saúde. 2010;**4**:649-658

[7] Oliveira F. Avaliação da força muscular e da contractura articular das mãos em pacientes com distrofia muscular de duchenne. Revista da Faculdade de medicina de Ribeirão Preto. 2010;**4**:65-78

[8] Nair S. Disabilities in children with Duchenne muscular dystrophy: A profile. Journal of Rehabilitation Medicine. 2001;**33**:147-149

[9] Mok E. Estimating body composition in children with Duchenne muscular dystrophy: Comparison of bioelectrical impedance analysis and skinfold-thickness measurement. The American Journal of Clinical Nutrition. 2006;(1):65-69

[10] Caromano A, Fátima L, Ana N, Ariane R, Érica N, Maria A, et al. Correlação entre massa de gordura corporal, força muscular, pressões respiratórias máximas e função na Distrofia Muscular de Duchenne. Conscientiae Saúde. 2010;**9**:10-18

[11] Pérez E. A eficácia da Hidrocinesioterapia em Crianças com Mielomeningocele Baixa. Brasil: Edições Cabo Frio; 2007

[12] Ortiz B. Hidroterapia nas disfunções que acometem crianças – Revisão bibliográfica. IX Encontro Latino Americano de Pós-Graduação. 3 a 5 de Setembro de 2011. Universidade do Vale do Paraíba, Brasil

[13] Campion M. Hidroterapia, Principios e Práticas. Brasil: Edições Sprint; 2000

[14] Fernandes L. Elaboração e Validação de Protocolos de Avaliação Funcional Para Portadores de DMD. Brasil: Edições Capes, Ciências da Reabilitação; 2006

[15] Vignos P. Management of progressive muscular dystrophy in childhood. Journal of the American Medical Association. 1963;**8**:103-112

[16] Christopher K. Neurodevelopmental needs in young boys with Duchenne muscular dystrophy (DMD): Observations from the cooperative

international neuromuscular research group (CINRG) DMD natural history study (DNHS). Plos Currents. 2018;**10**:1-18

[17] Yakimovich T, Kofman J, Lemaire E. Design and evaluation of a stance-control knee-ankle- foot orthosis knee joint. IEEE Transactions on Neural Systems and Rehabilitation Engineering. 2006;**14**:361-369

[18] Swan-Guerrero S. Potential Benefits of Exercise. College of Applied Health Sciences—Department of Disability and Human Development. Chicago, USA: UIC; 2007

Chapter 7

Pharmacological Actions and Potential Therapeutic Use of Cannabinoids in Duchenne's Muscular Dystrophy

Fabio Arturo Iannotti

Abstract

The scientific community uses the term endocannabinoid system (ECS) to refer to a large group of molecules that in our body control the production and function of the two major cannabinoid lipid mediators, namely, anandamide (AEA) and 2-arachidonoylglycerol (2-AG). Following their discovery, an impressive number of studies have shown that both AEA and 2-AG play a key role in a large plethora of functions in living organisms. Consequently, functional impairment or dysregulation of AEA and 2-AG activity leads to a variety of disorders affecting the nervous system as well as peripheral organs and tissues. For this reason, cannabinoids and/or cannabinoid synthetic drugs currently represent an important area of research for their potential therapeutic use to treat many human diseases having or not a genetic component. Despite these evidences, the role of the endocannabinoid system and hence potential changes in its activity in inherited muscular dystrophies remains largely unknown. Only recently, the role of endocannabinoid CB1 receptors was identified in Duchenne's muscular dystrophy (DMD). In this chapter, I summarize the chemical properties and functional role of the endocannabinoids as well as plant-derived cannabinoids during skeletal muscle formation and repair under physiological conditions as well as DMD.

Keywords: endocannabinoid system (ECS), endocannabinoids (ECs), cannabidiol (CBD), cannabidivarin (CBDV), cannabinoid receptor of type 1 (CB1), Duchenne's muscular dystrophy (DMD), transient receptor potential cation channels (TRP channels), anandamide (AEA), 2-arachidonoylglycerol (2-AG)

1. Introduction

1.1 Description of the endocannabinoid system (ECS)

The term endocannabinoid system (ECS) was originally coined in the 1990s after the discovery of brain receptors, responsive to Δ9-tetrahydrocannabinol-THC (the primary psychoactive substance of *Cannabis sativa*) and the class of their endogenous ligands identified immediately thereafter [1]. Since these discoveries, the number of molecules functionally associated with the activity of the endocannabinoid system has grown exponentially.

 IntechOpen

Nowadays, the ECS is considered to be a very complex network of connected signaling molecules, and key components of this system include (a) the two most potent endogenous agonists of cannabinoid receptors, anandamide (AEA) and 2-arachidonoyl-glycerol (2-AG), also named endocannabinoids; (b) endocannabinoid-related molecules including N-oleoylethanolamine (OEA) and N-palmitoylethanolamide (PEA); (c) the enzymes regulating the endocannabinoid biosynthesis (NAPE-PLD, ABDH4, GDE1, PTPN22 for AEA, and DAGLα and DAGLβ for 2-AG) and degradation (FAAH for AEA and MAGL, ABDH6, ABDH12, and FAAH for 2-AG); (d) the two endocannabinoids responsive to G-protein-coupled receptors known as cannabinoid receptor of type 1 (CB1) and type 2 (CB2); and (e) the cation permeant transient receptor potential vanilloid type-1 (TRPV1) [2–4]. Recently, AEA and 2-AG were also shown to have affinity for non-cannabinoid receptors including GABA-A, PPARγ, adenosine A3, and GPR55 [5]. In this complex scenario, also other endogenous AEA and 2-AG analogues, including other N-acyl-ethanolamines (NAEs), monoacylglycerols, N-acyl amino acids, and N-acyl-dopamines/taurines/serotonins, were suggested to share, to some extent, either anabolic or catabolic pathways, or both, with endocannabinoids (**Figure 1**) [6].

As also mentioned previously, the endocannabinoid system (ECS) is critically involved in regulating a variety of metabolic and cognitive processes. An overactive endocannabinoid/CB1R system has been associated with the development of obesity, insulin resistance, and dyslipidemia [7–10] as well as during the progression of neurological disorders such as Alzheimer's disease, multiple sclerosis, amyotrophic

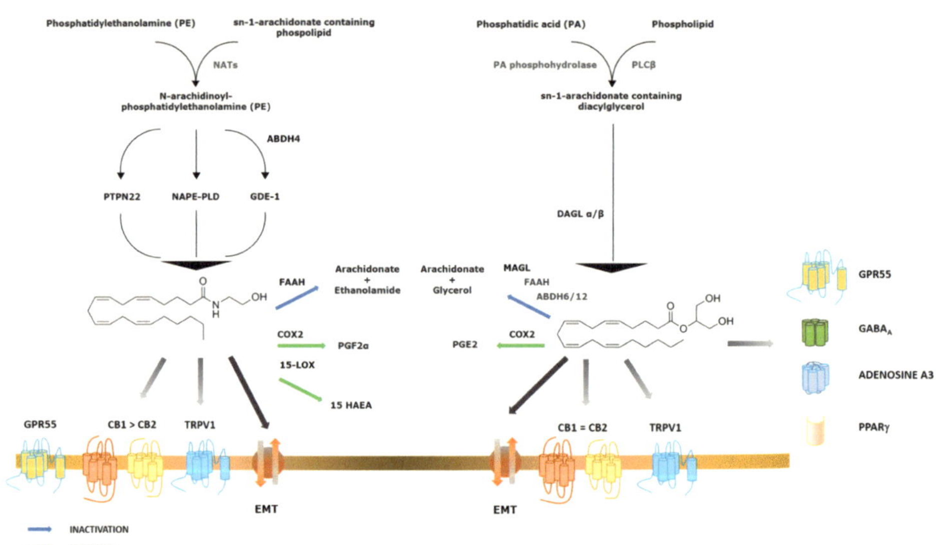

Figure 1.
Synthesis, inactivation, and mechanism of action of the two endocannabinoids anandamide and 2-AG. Thick black arrows indicate the biochemical reactions that starting from the precursor membranes lead to the synthesis of the two endocannabinoids anandamide and 2AG. ABDH4, α β-hydrolase 4; ABDH6, α β-hydrolase 6; ABDH12, α β-hydrolase 12; CB1 and CB2, cannabinoid receptor of types 1 and 2; COX2, cyclooxygenase 2; DAG, diacylglycerol; EMT, endocannabinoid membrane transporter; FAAH, fatty acid amide hydrolase; GDE1, glycerophosphodiester phosphodiesterase 1; MAGL, monoacylglycerol lipase; NAPE-PLD, N-acyl-phosphatidylethanolamine-selective phosphodiesterase; NATs, N-acyltransferases; PA, phosphatidic acid; PLCbeta, phospholipase Cbeta; PLD, phospholipase D; 15-LOX, 15-lipoxygenase; PTPN22, protein tyrosine phosphatase, non-receptor type 22; PGF2α, prostaglandin F2alpha; 15 HAEA, 15(S)-HETE ethanolamide; PGE2, prostaglandin E2; TRPV1, transient receptor potential, vanilloid subtype 1 receptor (this figure was copied directly from Arturo, Iannotti Fabio, and Fabiana, Piscitelli (Nov. 2018) Endocannabinoidome. In: eLS. John Wiley & Sons Ltd, Chichester). http://www.els.net [doi: 10.1002/9780470015902.a0028301].

lateral sclerosis, Parkinson's disease, and Huntington's chorea [4, 11]. Nevertheless, the potential role of the ECS in skeletal muscle disorders remains largely unknown.

2. What is known about the role of endocannabinoid systems in skeletal muscle

2.1 The role of the endocannabinoid system on glucose metabolism and insulin sensitivity in skeletal muscles

The first evidence demonstrating that CB1 receptors are functionally expressed in skeletal muscle tissues came out in 2005, when Liu and colleagues reported the effects of SR141716 (commonly known as rimonabant), one of the most used selective CB1 antagonists/inverse agonists [12], on energy expenditure and glucose uptake in isolated soleus muscle of obese *Lep(ob)/Lep(ob)* mice. In particular, the authors found that 5 days after daily treatment, SR141716 resulted in a significant reduction of daily food intake and body weight. While after 7 days, SR141716 had also positive effects on basal oxygen consumption and glucose uptake [13].

Few years later, Cavuoto and colleagues in two parallel studies demonstrated first that not only CB1 but also CB2, TRPV1, and FAAH are expressed in human and rodent skeletal muscle. Then, in human primary myotubes isolated from lean and obese donors, they found that the exposure to AEA or AM251 (another largely used selective CB1 antagonist), separately or in combination for 24 hours, induces significant changes in transcript levels of key genes regulating the metabolism such as AMP-activated protein kinase (AMPK) alpha 1 (alpha1) and alpha 2 (alpha2), pyruvate dehydrogenase kinase 4 (PDK4), and peroxisome proliferator-activated receptor-gamma coactivator-1alpha (PGC-1alpha) [14, 15].

Thus, these pioneering studies have paved the way for other studies through which the role of the ECS in regulating energy balance at the skeletal muscle level was further strengthened. In this regard, Esposito and colleagues showed that in differentiated L6 myotubes, the pharmacological blockade by SR141716 or genetic silencing of CB1 small interfering RNA sequences increased 2-deoxy-glucose uptake (2-DG) in a time- and dose-dependent manner. The authors also demonstrated that, the activity of phosphatidylinositol-3-kinase (PI3K) that in turn has stimulatory effects phosphoinositide-dependent kinase 1, Akt/protein kinase B, and protein kinase Cζ, resulted increased by SR141716 [16]. Accordingly, Eckardt et al. found that in human skeletal muscle cells 24 hours of incubation with adipocyte-conditioned medium (CM) or anandamide (AEA) impaired insulin-stimulated Akt(Ser473) phosphorylation. By contrast, pretreatment with rimonabant or AM251 reduced the effect of CM by about one-half, while the effect of AEA was fully prevented. The reduction of insulin-stimulated glucose uptake by CM was completely prevented by rimonabant. In addition, AEA was found to transiently activate ERK1/ERK2 and p38 mitogen-activated protein kinase and impaired insulin-stimulated Akt (Ser473) phosphorylation, but had no effect on Akt (Thr308) and glycogen synthase kinase 3 alpha/beta phosphorylation. Surprisingly, after 24 hours of treatment, an enhanced IRS-1 (Ser307) phosphorylation induced by AEA was observed in human skeletal muscle cells [17]. Furthermore, activation or inhibition of CB1 receptor activity exerts a differential effect with regard to MAP kinase- and PKB-directed signaling [18]. In conclusion, all these studies provide robust evidence that the endocannabinoid "tone" (hence CB1 signaling) is dysregulated during the obesity where its overactivity generates detrimental consequences on insulin sensitivity and consequently glucose catabolism in skeletal muscle cells.

It is worth noticing, however, that there are some discrepancies in scientific literature on whether the stimulation or inhibition of CB1 receptors has positive or negative effects on glucose metabolism in skeletal muscles. These differences are likely due to the dose/concentration and incubation time of agonists and antagonists of CB1 or more simply to the experimental model used. For a more extensive overview on the results aforementioned, Heyman et al. have recently published an extensive literature review [19].

2.2 Changes in the ECS activity in response to physical exercise

In addition to the diet, the physical exercise also contributes to induce changes in ECS activity. In this regard, Sparling et al. were the first in 2003 to find a robust increase of AEA in plasma of young male volunteers subjected to a physical exercise of moderate intensity. This trend of increase, but much less prominent, was observed also for 2-AG [20]. Other studies have further demonstrated the close relationship between the intensity and type of physical exercise and ECS activity. In particular, while an exercise of moderate intensity was confirmed to increase the plasma levels of AEA in human volunteers, surprisingly no changes in plasma ECs were observed following a very-high- and very-low-intensity exercise [21–23]. Of note, the increased ECS activity induced by exercise was positively correlated with the beneficial antidepressant effects of exercise at central as well as peripheral levels including sense of well-being, anxiety reduction, postexercise calm, and reduced pain sensation [20, 23–26]. Interestingly, Hill et al. found that augmentation of exercise-induced increase of endocannabinoid tone suppresses stress-associated behaviors and promotes hippocampal cell proliferation, in a manner dependent on stimulation of CB1 stimulation [27, 28]. In addition, Heyman et al. provided evidence in humans that following acute exercise AEA and BDNF, a key neurotrophic factor regulating the brain development and cognitive functions [19], were positively correlated at the end of exercise and after the 15-min recovery.

As yet, the genetic deletion of CB receptors from the brain on VTA GABAergic neurons decreased wheel-running performance in mice [29]. However, quite surprisingly, when Gamelin et al. evaluated changes in the levels of AEA and 2-AG as well as of congener molecules in high-fat (HFD) diet subjected to 12 weeks of exercise training, they found that the high-fat diet paired with exercise training had no effect on AEA, 2-AG, and AEA congener levels nor in the hypothalamus or hippocampus. However, CB1 expression levels were significantly increased in the hippocampus in response to HFD, exercise, and the combination of both, strengthening evidence for EC signaling involvement in neuronal plasticity following diet and/or exercise [30]. A more recent study shows differences in the circulating levels of 2-AG and AEA between male and female mice or between lines of mice bred for high levels of voluntary exercise, when compared to their nonselected control lines [31]. An increased ECS activity was also recently found in skeletal muscles of mice subjected to muscle atrophy induced by mechanical unloading, most likely due to the disuse-induced muscle inflammation or the altered glycolytic flux [32].

2.3 Changes in the ECS during the skeletal muscle formation

In spite of the important role played by the ECS in regulating the insulin sensitivity and oxidation pathways in skeletal muscle cells, its potential involvement during skeletal muscle formation and regeneration is little known. In 2014, our research group has demonstrated for the first time that the 2-AG levels significantly declined after 3 days of murine C2C12 myoblasts exposure to differentiation media and remained reduced up to at least day 7 of the differentiation process. In contrast,

AEA was not significantly changed during the myotube formation. According to these results, we have also demonstrated that during myotube formation the expression profile of the entire class of genes involved in AEA synthesis and degradation was not significantly changed, whereas the expression of key genes regulating the 2-AG metabolism including Daglα and Magl was significantly decreased and increased, respectively. Of note, potential changes in the endogenous levels of AEA and 2-AG were also explored during the skeletal muscle formation in vivo. In this case, we found that the levels of AEA were reduced in murine quadriceps muscle between the embryonic (E18) and early postnatal (P4) conditions, to then rebound at postnatal day 14 (P14). On the other hand, 2-AG levels remained constant between the embryonic and early postnatal phases but then decreased by about 50% at P14. In summary, there is evidence that during myogenesis, occurring both in vitro or in vivo, the endogenous levels of 2-AG decline with myotube formation and muscle growth, respectively. By contrast, the levels of AEA did not during the myotube formation in vitro but undergo oscillatory variations during muscle formation in vivo [33].

Furthermore, by the use of both pharmacological tools and techniques of gene silencing, we demonstrated that in murine and human myoblasts as well as human primary satellite cells, the stimulation of CB1 receptors with either exogenous or endogenously cannabinoids promotes myoblasts proliferation and inversely inhibits their differentiation in mature myotubes [33]. As yet, the stimulation of CB1 inhibits the activity of K_v7 (or KCNQ) channels, a subclass of voltage-gated K^+ channels composed of five members ($K_v7.1$–$K_v7.5$) that once activated promote myogenesis [33–35].

It is worth noting that both proliferation and differentiation of muscle precursor cells are both processes that are found altered in Duchenne's muscular dystrophy, thus representing one of the most severe causes underlying an inefficient muscle tissue regeneration, thus contributing to disease etiology and progression [36–38].

2.4 The role of the endocannabinoid system in Duchenne's muscular dystrophy

Among the hereditary myopathies, Duchenne's muscle dystrophy (DMD) represents the most frequent one, affecting predominantly young boys with a frequency of approximately 1:3500. Mutations in the X-linked gene encoding for the structural protein dystrophin, which plays a key structural role by physically linking the cytoskeleton to the surrounding extracellular matrix through the cell membrane, are the cause of the disease. The most frequent mutation are large intragenic deletions (65% of the cases), intragenic duplications (6–10% of the cases), or point mutations associated to other sequence variations (30–35% of the cases). Dysfunctional dystrophin leads to progressive and irreversible loss of muscle function [39–42].

As briefly mentioned earlier, it has been recently demonstrated that the lack of functional dystrophin is also the primary cause of an asymmetric cell division, altered morphogenesis, and inefficient differentiation of satellite cells, the muscle stem cells normally deputed to regenerate injured muscle fibers [36, 38]. Surprisingly, the number of satellite cells was found significantly increased in both human and murine skeletal muscles affected by DMD. Thus, while at the early stage of DMD, satellite cell-mediated muscle regeneration is able to attenuate degeneration; at later stages of disease progression, this process is inefficient [37, 43].

Therefore, in the light of these findings as well as the prominent role played by ECS during skeletal muscle cell and proliferation earlier described, my research group has explored whether the cannabinoids might represent a promising alternative approach to treat skeletal muscle disorders including DMD.

Toward this goal, we have recently characterized the expression profile of the ECS in whole muscles and isolated myoblasts of both mice and patients affected by DMD. No statistically significant differences were found in 2-AG levels between healthy and DMD donors, while higher levels of 2-AG were found in the muscles of 3-weeks-old mdx mice. However, 2-AG levels in both mdx mouse quadriceps and gastrocnemius, and in control gastrocnemius, first decreased (from 3 to 5 weeks of age) and then increased (from 5 to 8 weeks of age). Interestingly, 2-AG levels in the gastrocnemius were higher in mdx mice at 8 weeks and then 3 and 5 weeks.

Furthermore, in agreement with previous studies [36, 37, 43], we found that the total number of satellite cells isolated from skeletal muscles of mdx mice was significantly higher than in control mice. Intriguingly, by means of quantitative qPCR (qPCR) and RNA-Seq analysis, we demonstrated that the lack of dystrophin was accompanied by a significant increase in the transcript levels of CB1, occurring exclusively in satellite cells but not in other muscle resident cells including fibro-adipogenic progenitor (FAP) or macrophage cells. Thus, we provided evidence that in both human and murine skeletal muscles affected by DMD occur significant changes in 2-AG levels. These changes are associated with an increased expression of CB1 gene and concomitant increase in the number of satellite cells [44].

In addition to these findings, we have also demonstrated that PAX7, the most known master gene regulating satellite cell activation and self-renewal [45, 46], underwent changes very similar to CB1 showing a bell-shaped profile with the highest degree of expression at DMD onset and declining then over time. Intriguingly, by the use of bioinformatics and biochemical analyses, it was demonstrated that PAX7 directly binds and upregulates the CB1 gene in dystrophic more than in healthy muscles. In summary, the incorrect PAX7-CB1 cross talk, causing an excessive satellite cell proliferation and reduction of differentiation, was uncovered as a new target mechanism to treat DMD. Antagonism of CB1 receptors by rimonabant, opposite to their activation by ACEA, reduces human satellite cell proliferation and enhances the formation of myotubes from either satellite cells from healthy tissue or human myoblasts from DMD patients. Furthermore, in dystrophic mdx mice, the acute (2 weeks) or prolonged (12 weeks) treatment with rimonabant significantly prevented the loss of muscle coordination and strength compared to control (not treated) mice. Biochemical and histological analyses of mdx mice at the end of treatment revealed that the effect of rimonabant was associated with an increased number of healthy/regenerating fibers and decreased tissue levels of inflammatory markers including interleukin-6 receptor (IL-6R), tumor necrosis factor-α (TNFα), transforming growth factor β (TGF-β), and inducible nitric oxide synthase (iNOS) (**Figure 2**).

2.5 The use of plant-derived cannabinoids in Duchenne's muscular dystrophy

In addition to endocannabinoids, our research group has also explored the use of plant-derived cannabinoids (or phytocannabinoids) to treat DMD. Phytocannabinoids encompass a group of numerous compounds present in *Cannabis sativa.* Due to its euphoric properties, Δ^9-tetrahydrocannabinol (THC) is the best-known constituent of *Cannabis* [47]. However, many other phytocannabinoids (more than 100) have been purified and chemically characterized [48]. Among them, cannabidiol (CBD) and its analog cannabivarin (CBDV), contrary to Δ^9-THC, do not induce euphoric effects and showed their efficacy in a considerable number of preclinical as well as clinical studies [49–52]. Besides CBD and CBDV, *Cannabis sativa* may also contain up to 50% of Δ^9-tetrahydrocannabivarin (THCV), the propyl side chain analog of THC ([53, 54]. THCV is also undergoing clinical evaluation for the treatment of metabolic disorders [55]. In differentiating

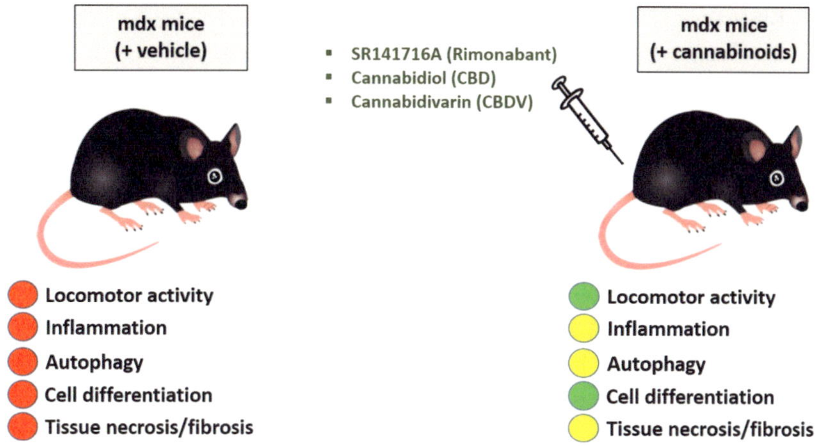

Figure 2.
Graphical representation showing the effects of cannabinoids in mdx mice.

C2C12 myoblasts, we found that the CBD (1 μM) and CBDV (1 and 3 μM), but not THCV, significantly promoted the myotube formation. Intriguingly, this latter effect was more pronounced following acute (5, 15 min and 3 hours) rather than the prolonged (72 hours) exposure and associated with a transient elevation of $[Ca^{2+}]_i$ in a manner dependent on TRPV1 channel activation. The efficacy of CBD and CBDV has been then demonstrated in vivo. In mdx mice of 5 weeks, the most used animal model of DMD [56, 57], we found that the locomotor activity measured by means of three different tests (rotarod, weight, and forelimb grip strength) was rescued completely when compared to control vehicle-treated mice. Of note, the effect of CBD and CBDV in mdx mice was not only found at 7 weeks (a time near the disease onset) but also at 34 weeks, when the muscle damage had further progressed. Interestingly, the beneficial effects of the phytocannabinoids were associated with a local or systemic anti-inflammatory effect and restoration of autophagy, two pathophysiological features of DMD (**Figure 2**) [36, 58]. However, in our recent published study, we did not perform a detailed time-course experiments; therefore, we cannot draw any conclusion as to whether the anti-inflammatory effects of the phytocannabinoids are the cause or the consequence of their pro-autophagic actions nor on whether at different stages of the disease; these compounds may affect myoblast differentiation. On the other hand, the finding of their anti-inflammatory and pro-autophagic actions opens the possibility of testing CBD and CBDV as add-on therapeutics to other agents that are currently undergoing clinical trials in DMD, such as exon-skipping agents [59]. However, it is worth mentioning that mdx mice do not model appropriately all aspects of the human DMD disease. Therefore, while beyond the scope of the present investigation, future studies in more suitable models, such as the golden retriever dog model [56, 57], are needed in order to suggest the therapeutic use of CBD and CBDV in DMD. In primary human satellite cells, CBD and CBDV and also THCV were capable of enhancing differentiation. Most importantly similar were also obtained in differentiating myoblasts isolated from seven different donors (ranging from 1 to 7 years old) diagnosed with DMD. Thus, these results potentially extended the therapeutic usefulness of these compounds at counteracting dystrophies. Interestingly, in satellite cells, the target through which these compounds produce their differentiating effect appears to be different from that mediating this effect in murine C2C12 myoblasts. In fact, TRPA1, rather than TRPV1, channels mediated an elevation of $[Ca^{2+}]_i$.

3. Conclusions

Inherited muscular dystrophies originating from mutations in one of the components forming the dystrophin glycoprotein complex show specific features but similar clinical characteristics. Albeit controversial, no overt clinical improvement was observed in patients with DMD under current therapies. For this reason, the identification of therapies capable of alleviating the progression of the disease is imperative. There are emerging evidences that the pharmacological regulation of ECS activity as well as the use of certain phytocannabinoids may attenuate the progressive and irreversible loss of muscle function. In conclusion, there is hope that the use of cannabinoids in DMD could represent a keystone to open new fields of research in discovering novel mechanisms able to preserve muscle tissue activity by preserving its integrity or promoting its regeneration.

Conflict of interest

I confirm there are no conflicts of interest.

Author details

Fabio Arturo Iannotti
Endocannabinoid Research Group, Institute of Biomolecular Chemistry (ICB), National Research Council (CNR), Pozzuoli, NA, Italy

*Address all correspondence to: fabio.iannotti@icb.cnr.it

References

[1] Di Marzo V, Bifulco M, De Petrocellis L. The endocannabinoid system and its therapeutic exploitation. Nature Reviews. Drug Discovery. 2004;**3**:771-784

[2] Di Marzo V, De Petrocellis L. Why do cannabinoid receptors have more than one endogenous ligand? Philosophical Transactions of the Royal Society of London. Series B, Biological Sciences. 2012;**367**:3216-3228

[3] Iannotti FA, Piscitelli F, Martella A, Mazzarella E, Allarà M, Palmieri V, et al. Analysis of the & quot; endocannabinoidome& quot; in peripheral tissues of obese Zucker rats. Prostaglandins, Leukotrienes, and Essential Fatty Acids. 2013;**89**:127-135

[4] Iannotti FA, Di Marzo V, Petrosino S. Endocannabinoids and endocannabinoid-related mediators: Targets, metabolism and role in neurological disorders. Progress in Lipid Research. 2016;**62**:107-128

[5] Baggelaar MP, Maccarrone M, van der Stelt M. 2-Arachidonoylglycerol: A signaling lipid with manifold actions in the brain. Progress in Lipid Research. 2018;**71**:1-17

[6] Di Marzo V, Wang J. Endocannabinoidome: The World of Endocannabinoids and Related Mediators. Academic Press; 19 September 2014. ISBN: 9780128004296, ISBN: 9780124201262

[7] Gatta-Cherifi B, Cota D. New insights on the role of the endocannabinoid system in the regulation of energy balance. International Journal of Obesity. 2016;**40**:210-219

[8] Perkins JM, Davis SN. Endocannabinoid system overactivity and the metabolic syndrome: Prospects for treatment. Current Diabetes Reports. 2008;**8**:12-19

[9] Di Marzo V. CB1 receptor antagonism: Biological basis for metabolic effects. Drug Discovery Today. 2008;**13**:1026-1041

[10] Di Marzo V. The endocannabinoid system in obesity and type 2 diabetes. Diabetologia. 2008;**51**:1356-1367

[11] Bisogno T, Di Marzo V. Cannabinoid receptors and endocannabinoids: Role in neuroinflammatory and neurodegenerative disorders. CNS & Neurological Disorders Drug Targets. 2010;**9**:564-573

[12] Rinaldi-Carmona M, Barth F, Héaulme M, Shire D, Calandra B, Congy C, et al. SR141716A, a potent and selective antagonist of the brain cannabinoid receptor. FEBS Letters. 1994;**350**:240-244

[13] Liu YL, Connoley IP, Wilson CA, Stock MJ. Effects of the cannabinoid CB1 receptor antagonist SR141716 on oxygen consumption and soleus muscle glucose uptake in Lep ob/Lep ob mice. International Journal of Obesity. 2005;**29**:183-187

[14] Cavuoto P, McAinch AJ, Hatzinikolas G, Janovská A, Game P, Wittert GA. The expression of receptors for endocannabinoids in human and rodent skeletal muscle. Biochemical and Biophysical Research Communications. 2007;**364**:105-110

[15] Cavuoto P, McAinch AJ, Hatzinikolas G, Cameron-Smith D, Wittert GA. Effects of cannabinoid receptors on skeletal muscle oxidative pathways. Molecular and Cellular Endocrinology. 2007;**267**:63-69

[16] Esposito I, Proto MC, Gazzerro P, Laezza C, Miele C, Alberobello AT,

et al. The cannabinoid CB1 receptor antagonist rimonabant stimulates 2-deoxyglucose uptake in skeletal muscle cells by regulating the expression of phosphatidylinositol-3-kinase. Molecular Pharmacology. 2008;**74**:1678-1686

[17] Eckardt K, Sell H, Taube A, Koenen M, Platzbecker B, Cramer A, et al. Cannabinoid type 1 receptors in human skeletal muscle cells participate in the negative crosstalk between fat and muscle. Diabetologia. 2009;**52**:664-674

[18] Lipina C, Stretton C, Hastings S, Hundal JS, Mackie K, Irving AJ, et al. Regulation of MAP kinase-directed mitogenic and protein kinase B-mediated signaling by cannabinoid receptor type 1 in skeletal muscle cells. Diabetes. 2010;**59**:375-385

[19] Heyman E, Gamelin F-X, Aucouturier J, Di Marzo V. The role of the endocannabinoid system in skeletal muscle and metabolic adaptations to exercise: Potential implications for the treatment of obesity. Obesity Reviews. 2012;**13**:1110-1124

[20] Sparling PB, Giuffrida A, Piomelli D, Rosskopf L, Dietrich A. Exercise activates the endocannabinoid system. NeuroReport. 2003;**14**:2209-2211

[21] Feuerecker M, Hauer D, Toth R, Demetz F, Hölzl J, Thiel M, et al. Effects of exercise stress on the endocannabinoid system in humans under field conditions. European Journal of Applied Physiology. 2012;**112**:2777-2781

[22] Heyman E, Gamelin F-X, Goekint M, Piscitelli F, Roelands B, Leclair E, et al. Intense exercise increases circulating endocannabinoid and BDNF levels in humans—Possible implications for reward and depression. Psychoneuroendocrinology. 2012;**37**:844-851

[23] Raichlen DA, Foster AD, Seillier A, Giuffrida A, Gerdeman GL. Exercise-induced endocannabinoid signaling is modulated by intensity. European Journal of Applied Physiology. 2013;**113**:869-875

[24] Keeney BK, Meek TH, Middleton KM, Holness LF, Garland T. Sex differences in cannabinoid receptor-1 (CB1) pharmacology in mice selectively bred for high voluntary wheel-running behavior. Pharmacology, Biochemistry, and Behavior. 2012;**101**:528-537

[25] Dietrich A, McDaniel WF. Endocannabinoids and exercise. British Journal of Sports Medicine. 2004;**38**:536-541

[26] Keeney BK, Raichlen DA, Meek TH, Wijeratne RS, Middleton KM, Gerdeman GL, et al. Differential response to a selective cannabinoid receptor antagonist (SR141716: Rimonabant) in female mice from lines selectively bred for high voluntary wheel-running behaviour. Behavioural Pharmacology. 2008;**19**:812-820

[27] Hill MN, Titterness AK, Morrish AC, Carrier EJ, Lee TT-Y, Gil-Mohapel J, et al. Endogenous cannabinoid signaling is required for voluntary exercise-induced enhancement of progenitor cell proliferation in the hippocampus. Hippocampus. 2009;**20**:NA-NA

[28] Hill MN, Kambo JS, Sun JC, Gorzalka BB, Galea LAM. Endocannabinoids modulate stress-induced suppression of hippocampal cell proliferation and activation of defensive behaviours. The European Journal of Neuroscience. 2006;**24**:1845-1849

[29] Dubreucq S, Durand A, Matias I, Bénard G, Richard E, Soria-Gomez E, et al. Ventral tegmental area cannabinoid type-1 receptors control voluntary exercise performance. Biological Psychiatry. 2013;**73**:895-903

[30] Gamelin F-X, Aucouturier J, Iannotti FA, Piscitelli F, Mazzarella E,

Aveta T, et al. Exercise training and high-fat diet elicit endocannabinoid system modifications in the rat hypothalamus and hippocampus. Journal of Physiology and Biochemistry. 2016;**73**:335-347

[31] Thompson Z, Argueta D, Garland T, DiPatrizio N. Circulating levels of endocannabinoids respond acutely to voluntary exercise, are altered in mice selectively bred for high voluntary wheel running, and differ between the sexes. Physiology & Behavior. 2017;**170**:141-150

[32] Hutchins-Wiese HL, Li Y, Hannon K, Watkins BA. Hind limb suspension and long-chain omega-3 PUFA increase mRNA endocannabinoid system levels in skeletal muscle. The Journal of Nutritional Biochemistry. 2012;**23**:986-993

[33] Iannotti FA, Silvestri C, Mazzarella E, Martella A, Calvigioni D, Piscitelli F, et al. The endocannabinoid 2-AG controls skeletal muscle cell differentiation via CB1 receptor-dependent inhibition of Kv7 channels. Proceedings of the National Academy of Sciences of the United States of America. 2014;**111**:E2472-E2481

[34] Iannotti FA, Barrese V, Formisano L, Miceli F, Taglialatela M. Specification of skeletal muscle differentiation by repressor element-1 silencing transcription factor (REST)-regulated Kv7.4 potassium channels. Molecular Biology of the Cell. 2013;**24**:274-284

[35] Iannotti FA, Panza E, Barrese V, Viggiano D, Soldovieri MV, Taglialatela M. Expression, localization, and pharmacological role of Kv7 potassium channels in skeletal muscle proliferation, differentiation, and survival after myotoxic insults. The Journal of Pharmacology and Experimental Therapeutics. 2010;**332**:811-820

[36] Dumont NA, Wang YX, Von Maltzahn J, Pasut A, Bentzinger CF, Brun CE, et al. Dystrophin expression in muscle stem cells regulates their polarity and asymmetric division. Nature Medicine. 2015;**21**:1455-1463

[37] Kottlors M, Kirschner J. Elevated satellite cell number in Duchenne muscular dystrophy. Cell and Tissue Research. 2010;**340**:541-548

[38] Chang NC, Chevalier FP, Rudnicki MA. Satellite cells in muscular dystrophy-lost in polarity. Trends in Molecular Medicine. 2016;**22**:479-496

[39] Falzarano M, Scotton C, Passarelli C, Ferlini A. Duchenne muscular dystrophy: From diagnosis to therapy. Molecules. 2015;**20**:18168-18184

[40] Nallamilli BRR, Ankala A, Hegde M. Molecular diagnosis of duchenne muscular dystrophy. Current Protocols in Human Genetics. 2014;**83**: 9.25.1-9. 25.29

[41] Govoni A, Magri F, Brajkovic S, Zanetta C, Faravelli I, Corti S, et al. Ongoing therapeutic trials and outcome measures for Duchenne muscular dystrophy. Cellular and Molecular Life Sciences. 2013;**70**:4585-4602

[42] Magri F, Govoni A, D'Angelo MG, Del Bo R, Ghezzi S, Sandra G, et al. et al., Genotype and phenotype characterization in a large dystrophinopathic cohort with extended follow-up. Journal of Neurology. 2011;**258**:1610-1623

[43] Jiang C, Wen Y, Kuroda K, Hannon K, Rudnicki MA, Kuang S. Notch signaling deficiency underlies age-dependent depletion of satellite cells in muscular dystrophy. Disease Models & Mechanisms. 2014;**7**:997-1004

[44] Iannotti FA, Pagano E, Guardiola O, Adinolfi S, Saccone V, Consalvi S, et al. Genetic and pharmacological regulation

of the endocannabinoid CB1 receptor in Duchenne muscular dystrophy. Nature Communications. 2018;**9**:3950

[45] Seale P, Sabourin LA, Girgis-Gabardo A, Mansouri A, Gruss P, Rudnicki MA. Pax7 is required for the specification of myogenic satellite cells. Cell. 2000;**102**:777-786

[46] Reimann J, Brimah K, Schröder R, Wernig A, Beauchamp JR, Partridge TA. Pax7 distribution in human skeletal muscle biopsies and myogenic tissue cultures. Cell and Tissue Research. 2004;**315**:233-242

[47] Di Marzo V, Piscitelli F. The endocannabinoid system and its modulation by phytocannabinoids. Neurotherapeutics. 2015;**12**:692-698

[48] Morales P, Hurst DP, Reggio PH. Molecular targets of the phytocannabinoids: A complex picture. Progress in the Chemistry of Organic Natural Products. 2017;**103**:103-131

[49] Burstein SH, Zurier RB. Cannabinoids, endocannabinoids, and related analogs in inflammation. The AAPS Journal. 2009;**11**:109-119

[50] Hill AJ, Williams CM, Whalley BJ, Stephens GJ. Phytocannabinoids as novel therapeutic agents in CNS disorders. Pharmacology & Therapeutics. 2012;**133**:79-97

[51] Fernández-Ruiz J, Moro MA, Martínez-Orgado J. Cannabinoids in neurodegenerative disorders and stroke/brain trauma: From preclinical models to clinical applications. Neurotherapeutics. 2015;**12**:793-806

[52] Feliú A, Moreno-Martet M, Mecha M, Carrillo-Salinas FJ, de Lago E, Fernández-Ruiz J, et al. A Sativex ® -like combination of phytocannabinoids as a disease-modifying therapy in a viral model of multiple sclerosis. British Journal of Pharmacology. 2015;**172**:3579-3595

[53] Fischedick JT. Identification of terpenoid chemotypes among high (−)-trans-Δ9- tetrahydrocannabinol-producing *Cannabis sativa L. Cultivars*. Cannabis and Cannabinoid Research. 2017;**2**:34-47

[54] McPartland JM, Duncan M, Di Marzo V, Pertwee RG. Are cannabidiol and \$Δ\$(9) -tetrahydrocannabivarin negative modulators of the endocannabinoid system? A systematic review. British Journal of Pharmacology. 2015;**172**:737-753

[55] Jadoon KA, Ratcliffe SH, Barrett DA, Thomas EL, Stott C, Bell JD, et al. Efficacy and safety of cannabidiol and tetrahydrocannabivarin on glycemic and lipid parameters in patients with type 2 diabetes: A randomized, double-blind, placebo-controlled, parallel group pilot study. Diabetes Care. 2016;**39**:1777-1786

[56] Collins CA, Morgan JE. Duchenne's muscular dystrophy: Animal models used to investigate pathogenesis and develop therapeutic strategies. International Journal of Experimental Pathology. 2003;**84**:165-172

[57] McGreevy JW, Hakim CH, McIntosh MA, Duan D. Animal models of Duchenne muscular dystrophy: From basic mechanisms to gene therapy. Disease Models & Mechanisms. 2015;**8**:195-213

[58] Fiacco E, Castagnetti F, Bianconi V, Madaro L, De Bardi M, Nazio F, et al. Autophagy regulates satellite cell ability to regenerate normal and dystrophic muscles. Cell Death and Differentiation. 2016;**23**:1839-1849

[59] Nakamura A. Moving towards successful exon-skipping therapy for Duchenne muscular dystrophy. Journal of Human Genetics. 2017;**62**:871-876

Section 5

The Muscular Dystrophy Model

Chapter 8

Interspecies Translation: Bovine Marbling to Human Muscular Dystrophy

Jose L. Valenzuela, Sally S. Lloyd, Edward J. Steele, Francis L. Mastaglia and Roger L. Dawkins

Abstract

There are interesting similarities and differences when comparing the histopathology of bovine marbling and human muscular dystrophy. At the simplest level, both conditions are characterized by genetically controlled and more or less inexorable replacement of muscle fibers with fat cells. At issue is whether an improved understanding of these two processes can lead to better outcomes for patients. There are many forms of dystrophy that differ in their genetics and their histopathology. There are also many forms of "marbling" ranging from the coarse to fine, epimysial, perimysial to endomysial and even to total replacement or steatosis. A detailed examination of marbling will provide a framework for further investigation of human dystrophy. Ultimately, the many genetic factors involved can be addressed through a better understanding of the metabolic pathways involved in marbling.

Keywords: synteny, muscular dystrophy, bovine marbling, adipogenesis

1. Introduction

The purpose of this review is to compare the genetics and histopathology of bovine marbling and human muscular dystrophy. Surprisingly, in spite of similarities, the literature suggests that marbling is a function of extreme adipogenesis whereas dystrophy is a consequence of fundamental defects in muscle itself. In fact, completely independent studies, as summarized here, reveal that similar genes have been implicated in some selected situations. Further, it is clear that the histopathology of some forms of dystrophy can resemble some forms of bovine marbling.

2. Marbling

Marbling is the term used to describe the presence of macroscopically visible fat within muscle (**Figures 1** and **2**). Coarse marbling refers to white areas of fat through and around muscle bundles, generally as continuous bands arising from the subcutaneous adipose tissue. By contrast, fine or "snowflake" marbling is characterized by more even white flecks resulting in pink rather than red muscle.

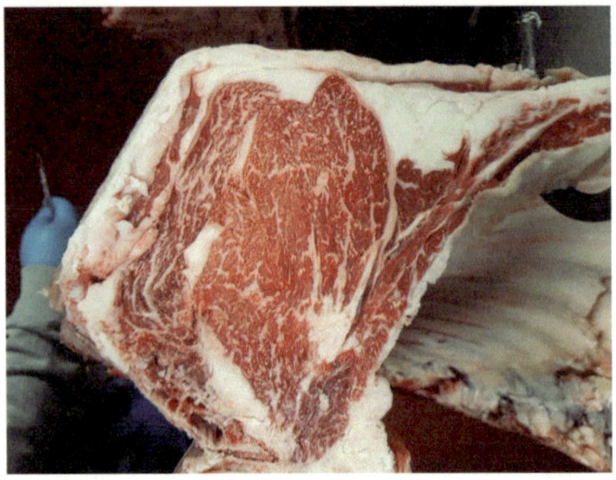

Figure 1.
Loin at the eleventh intercostal level of carcass of Melaleuka Stud steer M508 (wy63 ak25 dx13), MSA MB 1100, DOF 471. There are extensive areas of fine marbling as indicated by pink muscle with fine flecks. Note 88% Wagyu (63% black, 25% red). See also ***Figure 5*** *for microscopic features.*

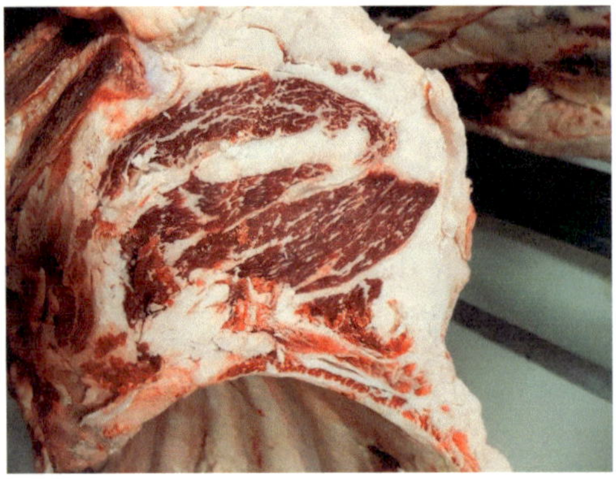

Figure 2.
Loin at the eleventh intercostal level of carcass of Melaleuka Stud heifer M621 (wy75 dx25), MSA MB 920, DOF 443. There is a predominance of fat arborizing from the subcutaneous tissue and creating coarse marbling. The muscle areas are dark red in comparison to ***Figure 1****. Note lower MSA MB of 920 but similar days on feed (DOF).*

These two forms may coexist but can be distinguished and quantified by skilled observers. Fine marbling is associated with improved taste and tenderness [1]. Further, it has been shown to relate to a preferred fatty acid profile. Accordingly, there is copious funding and now a substantial understanding of the environmental and genetic factors which favor fine rather than coarse.

3. Interspecies translation

Interspecies translation from cattle to man has unrecognized potential. Firstly, cattle are close to humans in evolutionary time and fall within that window of 50–100 million years of separation (or last common ancestor) which is characterized by very similar proteins but vastly different regulations of expression. The same window may explain the fact that the two species have synergized over some 40,000 years of contact and at least 7000 years of domestication. As one example, infections can be similar and, in some cases, are transmissible from one to the other, but close exposure to cattle is generally innocuous implying some form of immunity. As for example in the case of pox and tuberculosis. We argue that cattle are both relevant and relatively safe for translational studies.

Secondly, domestic cattle are well maintained, closely observed, and very well understood. There are huge databases and DNA banks which have been in existence for 50 years. Innumerable breeds can be compared often under different environmental conditions. Many of these breeds have been closed for hundreds of years and then intentionally crossed with each other. There is great potential for meaningful studies of population genetics and family and haplotype associations and, even more so, for structure-function genomics. Metabolic and inflammatory pathways are relatively well understood and are supported by inestimable funding available to ensure future supplies of meat, milk, cheese, butter, leather, and fertilizer.

Thirdly, cattle are plentiful and even more so than humans. Because the generation time and life expectancy are much shorter, there are excellent opportunities to study and treat genetically determined diseases prospectively [2].

4. Other instances of translation

White muscle disease or selenium/vitamin E deficiency occurs quite commonly in livestock raised on leached soils. The pathology resembles dystrophy in some respects. A mutation in the selenoprotein N gene (SEPN1) is responsible for some types of congenital muscular dystrophies and myopathies [3]. Kakulas [4] demonstrated that dystrophy-like changes explained the weakness observed in quokkas on Rottnest Island. Importantly, the condition could be corrected by treating the deficiency raising the possibility that human dystrophies could be reversible if the basic defect could be corrected.

5. Genomic approach

The term genome is used here to refer to the architecture of DNA sequences, whereas others have come to use the term in the context of single-nucleotide polymorphisms wherever they occur. The difference is fundamental to the discovery of gene clusters with coherent cis and trans interactions between conserved sequences known as ancestral haplotypes [5–9]. Many studies have shown that the SNP approach in livestock and humans fails to identify these critical sequences and can be misleading at best [10]. SNPs are neutral markers of parentage rather than functionally important [11].

One major benefit of ancestral haplotypes as opposed to SNPs is that it is possible to use interspecies translation. During mammalian evolution, polymorphic frozen blocks have diverged to some extent although the functionally important sequences tend to be conserved.

As shown in **Figure 3** and **Table 1**, there are similarities between genomic regions on Hosa 17 and Bota 19. Although there have been architectural changes such as insertions and transversions, the gene content has been preserved.

Bota 19 was chosen as the reference because of its critical role in determining the degree of marbling between individuals of a breed, F1 crosses and between breeds [5, 12–14].

Hosa 17 was chosen for comparison because it contains some of the same genes such as TCAP. Further analysis revealed an extraordinary degree of preservation or synteny in spite of an evolutionary separation time of at least 50 million years and therefore millions of generations. Implicit is that there are functional reasons for similarities in genomic architecture.

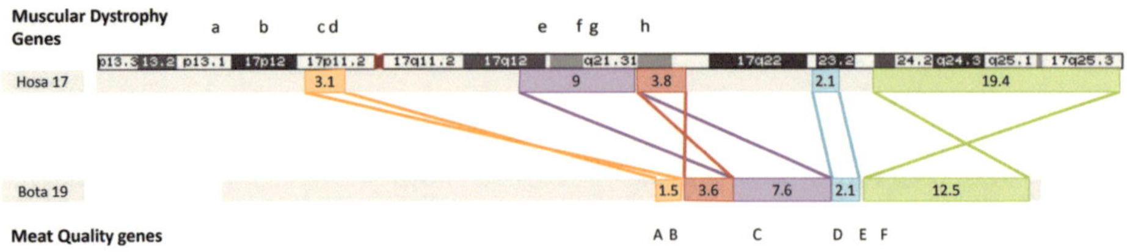

Figure 3.
Marbling and muscular dystrophy are syntenic on bovine chromosome 19 (Bota 19) and human chromosome 17 (Hosa 17). Colored boxes represent segments with the same gene content. Crossed joining lines indicate inverted translocations. Numbers represent Mb. Synteny was determined by the positions of homologous genes in the human assembly Hg 38 and bovine assembly BosTau8 located using the UCSC genome browser. Inverted sections and the exact location of boundaries between blocks were determined by dotplots comparing the two sequences. Adapted from: [13] Locations of ***Muscular Dystrophy Genes:*** *(a) MYH2, (b) PMP22, (c) TRPV2, (d) SREBF1, (e) TCAP, (f) CAVIN1, (g) BECN1, (h) SGCA and* ***Meat Quality Genes*** *(A)SREBF1, (B) MPRIP, (C) TCAP, (D) GH, (E) UTS2R, (F) FASN shown here. See* ***Table 1*** *for more information about these genes.*

Gene location	Description	Human muscular dystrophy	Meat quality trait
MYH2 Hosa 17p13.1 Bota chr19: 30.13Mb	MYH2 encodes the myosin heavy chain isoform that is expressed in fast type 2A muscle fibers	Proximal myopathy and ophthalmoplegia is caused by heterozygous, compound heterozygous, or homozygous mutation in MYH2 leading to a lack of type 2a fibres [18]	In pork, IMF, water holding capacity, and meat color [19]
PMP22 Hosa 17p12 Bota chr19: 33.35Mb	Peripheral myelin protein-22	Duplication of peripheral myelin protein 22 causes Charcot-Marie-Tooth disease type 1A [20]	
TRPV2 Hosa 17p11.2 Bota chr19: 33.816Mb	Transient receptor potential cation channel, V2: responds to heat and cations	Muscular dystrophy is ameliorated in dystrophin-deficient mdx mice by dominant-negative inhibition of TRPV2 [21]	
SREBF1 Hosa 17p11.2 Bota chr19: 35.23Mb	Sterol regulatory element-binding protein-1 controls cholesterol homeostasis by stimulating transcription of sterol-regulated genes	Mutations of LMNA that cause Emery-Dreifuss muscular dystrophy (EDMD2-AD) and familial partial lipodystrophy (FPLD2) result in less binding of lamin A to SREBP1 [22]	SREBF1 is involved in adipogenesis and polymorphisms are associated with fatty acid composition of Japanese Black Cattle [23]
MPRIP Hosa 17p11.2 Bota chr19: 35.557Mb	Myosin phosphatase rho-interacting protein targets myosin phosphatase to regulate the phosphorylation of myosin light chain [24]		Haplotypes diffentiated by polymorphsims in MRIP are associated with differences in intramuscular fat development in Wagyu [25]
SGCA Hosa 17q21.33 Bota chr19: 37.11Mb	Sarcoglycan, alpha Sarcoglycans form part of the dystrophin-glycoprotein complex	Mutations in SGCA cause limb-girdle muscular dystrophy type 2D. SGCB, SGCD, and SGCG are associated with LGMD types 2E, 2F, and 2C, respectively [26]	
TCAP Hosa 17q12 Bota chr19: 40.69Mb	Titin-cap (telethonin) is a sarcomeric protein localized to the periphery of Z discs that define the border of the sarcomere as a structural anchor and signaling center	Limb-girdle muscular dystrophy type 2G (LGMD2G) is caused by mutations in the TCAP gene [27]	A polymorphism of TCAP is associated with IMF content and fatty acid composition of beef [13, 28]

Gene location	Description	Human muscular dystrophy	Meat quality trait
CAVIN1 Hosa 17q21.2 Bota chr19: 43.14Mb	Cavin is an essential factor in the biogenesis of caveolae	Congenital generalized lipodystrophy, type 4; (CGL4) is caused by mutations in CAVIN1 that result in CAV 3 deficiency [29]	
BECN1 Hosa 17q21.31 Bota chr19: 43.47Mb	Beclin-1 participates in the regulation of autophagy	Expression of BECN1 was reduced in patients with muscular dystrophies BTHLM1 and UMCD1 which were caused by COL6A1 mutations [30]	Involved in proteolysis and beef aging [31]
GH1 Hosa 17q23.3 Bota Chr19: 48.77Mb	Growth Hormone		A polymorphism of growth hormone is associated with fatty acid composition of Wagyu beef [32]
FASN Hosa 17q25.3 Bota Chr19: 51.38 Mb	Fatty Acid Synthase the key enzyme of de novo lipogenesis to produce saturated fatty acids		Fatty Acid Synthase is highlighted in GWAS for fatty acid content and composition of Wagyu and Hanwoo beef [33, 34]
UTS2R Hosa17q25.3 Bota Chr19: 50.81 Mb	A receptor abundant in heart and pancreas and responsive to Urotensin II which has potent vasoactive properties		A polymorphism of UTS2R is associated with IMF content of Wagyu x Holstein beef [39]

Table 1.
Details of relevant genes in Bota 19 and Hosa 17.

Yet further analysis suggests some explanations for the co-location of similar genes. Irrespective of cis and trans interactions between the protein products, there is evidence of co-regulation (see, e.g., SREBP). In this context, we conclude that, although products and their regulating transcription factors are preserved, separation has permitted the insertion of species-specific elements, which control the quantitative differences between humans and cattle.

Importantly, as shown in **Figure 3** and **Table 1**, Hosa 17 contains multiple candidates for involvement in human muscular dystrophy. There is even more complexity in explaining the multiple candidates as shown in **Tables 2** and **3**.

Thus, syntenic analysis has suggested a novel approach to identification of operative elements in marbling and in some forms of dystrophy.

Gene location	Description	Human muscular dystrophy	Meat quality trait
MSTN Hosa 2q32.2 Bota chr2: 6.21Mb	Myostatin	Muscle hypertrophy was caused by a homozygous mutation in myostatin [35]	Mutations in myostatin cause double muscling in several cattle breeds [36]
CAPN3 Hosa 15q15.1 Bota chr10: 37.8Mb	Calpains are nonlysosomal intracellular cysteine proteases. CAPN3 is a muscle-specific large subunit	Limb-girdle muscular dystrophy type 2A (LGMD2A) is caused by homozygous or compound heterozygous mutation in CAPN3	SNPs within CAPN3 are associated with tenderness in *Bos Indicus* cattle [37]

Gene location	Description	Human muscular dystrophy	Meat quality trait
CAPN1 Hosa 11q13.1 Bota chr29: 44.06Mb	m-Calpain		Two CAPN1 genetic markers are associated with tenderness in Brahman beef [38]
DMD Hosa Xp21.2-.1 Bota chrX: 115.34Mb	Dystrophin maintains the structural integrity of myofibrils	Duchene muscular dystrophy	
LAMA2 Hosa 6q22.33 Bota chr9: 67.96Mb	LAMA2 gene encodes the alpha-2 chain of laminin-2 Laminin-2 (merosin) is the main laminin found in muscle fibers	Congenital merosin-deficient muscular dystrophy type 1A; MDC1A	
MYOT Hosa 5q31.2 Bota chr7: 50.94Mb	Myotilin directly binds F-actin and efficiently cross-links actin filaments and prevents filament disassembly	LGMD1A is caused by heterozygous mutation in the MYOT. It is characterized by adult-onset muscle weakness, progressing from the hip to the shoulder girdle	SNPs in MYOT correlate with loin muscle area and intramuscular fat in Qinchuan cattle[39]
CAV3 Hosa 3p25.3 Bota chr22: 17.83Mb	Caveolin 3	Muscular dystrophy, limb-girdle, type 1C; LGMD1C	
SGCD Hosa 5q33.2-.3 Bota chr7: 69.59Mb	Sarcoglycan, delta is expressed in skeletal and heart muscles and to a lesser extent in smooth muscle. Delta-sarcoglycan is localized at the sarcolemma	Muscular dystrophy, limb-girdle, type 2F; LGMD2F	
SGCE Hosa 7q21.3 Bota chr4: 11.84Mb	Epsilon-sarcoglycan	Myoclonus-dystonia is a genetically heterogeneous disorder characterized by myoclonic jerks affecting mostly proximal muscles	
SGCB Bota chr6: 69.53Mb	Beta-sarcoglycan		
SGCG at Bota chr12: 34.92Mb			
COL6A1 COL6A2 21q22.3	Collagen, type VI, alpha-1, and alpha-2 Members of the collagen VI family form distinct networks of microfibrils in connective tissue and interact with other extracellular matrix components	Ullrich congenital muscular dystrophy 1 Bethlem myopathy 1	
COL6A3 2q37.3	COLLAGEN, TYPE VI, ALPHA-3	Ullrich congenital muscular dystrophy 1, Bethlem myopathy 1 Dystonia 27	

DOI: http://dx.doi.org/10.5772/intechopen.82685

Gene location	Description	Human muscular dystrophy	Meat quality trait
ITGA7 12q13.2	The alpha-7 integrin is a specific cellular receptor for the basement membrane proteins laminin-1, laminin-2, and laminin-4. The alpha-7 subunit is expressed mainly in skeletal and cardiac muscles and may be involved in differentiation and migration processes during myogenesis	Congenital muscular dystrophy	
EMD Xq28	Emerin is found along the nuclear rim of many cell types and is a member of the nuclear lamina-associated protein family	Emery-dreifuss muscular dystrophy 1, X-LINKED; EDMD1	
ATP2A1 (SERCA-1) 16p11.2	Calcium-transporting ATPase lower cytoplasmic Ca(2+) concentration by pumping Ca(2+) to luminal or extracellular spaces. ATP2A1 is the ATPase type found in fast twitch muscles	Brody myopathy	
DES 2q35	Desmin is the muscle-specific member of the intermediate filament (IF) protein family. It is one of the earliest myogenic markers, both in the heart and somites, and is expressed in satellite stem cells and replicating myoblasts	Myopathy, myofibrillar, 1	
PLEC 8q24.3	Plectin-1 is one of the largest polypeptides known and is believed to provide mechanical strength to cells and tissues by acting as a cross-linking element of the cytoskeleton	Epidermolysis bullosa with muscular dystrophy Limb-girdle type 2Q	

Table 2.
Details of relevant genes outside of Hosa 17/Bota 19.

Absent protein	Dystrophy type	Gene location
Dystrophin	Xp21 muscular dystrophies (Duchenne, Becker)	DMD Hosa Xp21.2 p21.1 Bota chrX: 115,342,323-117,606,340
Sarcoglycans	Limb-girdle muscular dystrophies 2C-F	SGCA Hosa 17q21.33 Bota 19 SGCB Bota chr6 SGCD Hosa 5q33.2 Bota 7 SGCE Hosa 7q21.3 Bota 4 SGCG Bota chr12
Dysferlin	Limb-girdle muscular dystrophy 2B	DYSF Hosa 2p13.2
Caveolin-3	Limb-girdle muscular dystrophy 1a, rippling muscle disease, hyperCKemia	CAV3 Hosa 3p25.3 Bota 22 CAVIN1 Hosa 17q21.2 Bota 19
Telethonin	Limb-girdle muscular dystrophy 2G	TCAP Hosa 17q12 Bota 19
Laminin a2	MDC1A ("merosin"-deficient congenital muscular dystrophy)	LAMA2 Hosa 6q22.33, Bota 9
Collagen VI	Ullrich congenital muscular dystrophy	COL6A1&2 Hosa 21q22.3 COL6A3 Hosa 2q37.3
Integrin alpha7	Mild congenital dystrophy/myopathy	ITGA7 Hosa 12q13.2

Absent protein	Dystrophy type	Gene location
Calpain-3 (easier to assess on immunoblots than sections)	Limb-girdle muscular dystrophy 2A	CAPN3 Hosa 15q15.1 Bota 10
Emerin	X-Linked emery-dreifuss muscular dystrophy	EMD Hosa Xq28
SERCA 1	Brody disease	***ATP2A1 Hosa 16p11.2***
Plectin	Epidermolysis bullosa with muscular dystrophy, limb-girdle dystrophy 2Q	PLEC Hosa 8q24.3
LAMP-2	Danon disease	LAMP2 Xq24
Accumulating protein	**Dystrophy type**	**Gene location**
Actin	Congenital actin myopathy/nemaline myopathy	ACTA1 Hosa 1q24.13 TPM3 Hosa 1q23
Myosin	Myosin storage myopathy	MYH7 Hosa 14q11
Myotilin	Myotilin-related myofibrillar myopathy	MYOT Hosa 5q31.2
Desmin	Desmin myopathy	DES Hosa 2q35 SEPN1 Hosa 1p36

(Adapted from [15] Table 6.3 dystrophy related protein changes detectable with immunohistochemistry).

Table 3.
Protein accumulations and deficits in dystrophy.

6. Histopathological approach

The substantial range of changes found in the human dystrophies is illustrated in the study of Dubowitz et al. [15].

We are fortunate in having histological muscle samples from cattle with degrees of marbling [14]. Some of these changes are illustrated in **Figures 4–8** from three animals (M508, M621, and M129) fed a standard ration for 471, 443, and 481 days respectively. The macroscopic measure of marbling (MSA MB) ranged from high to moderate (1100, 920 and 820, respectively) as expected in high content Wagyu (88, 75, and 63%, respectively). A common feature is the invasion of adipose tissue between intact muscle fascicles (**Figure 4**). For the most part, the process extends along the perimysium leading to variation in fiber size, staining of myofibers (**Figures 5** and **6**), and the formation of residual islands of myofibers (**Figure 7**), which suggests an explanation for fine (see **Figure 1**) rather than coarse (see **Figure 2**) marbling; fine is due to more aggressive invasion reflecting quantitative differences in gene regulation.

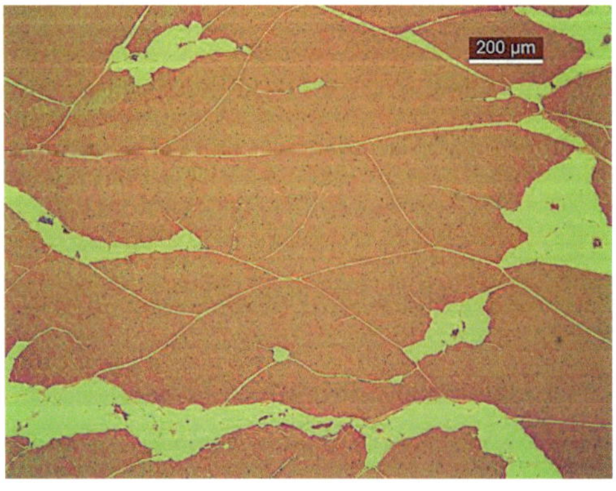

Figure 4.
*Highly marbled loin muscle shows a pattern of fat arborization and invasion with adipocytes predominantly in the perimysium, between muscle fascicles. Note extensive vascularization centrally within the fat. M508 (wy63 ak25 dx13), MSA MB 1100, DOF 471. See also **Figure 1**.*

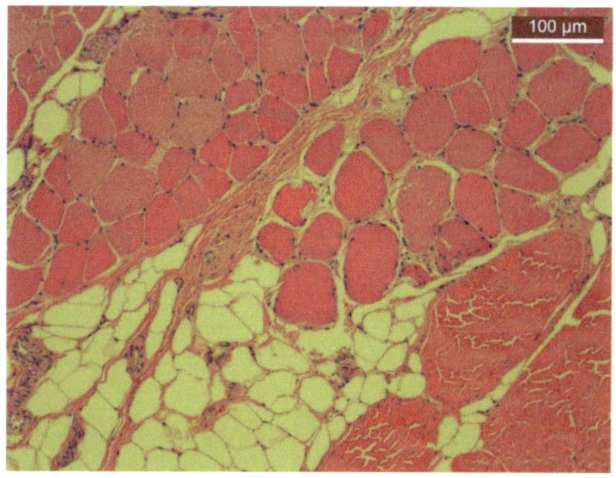

Figure 5.
Histological section of Sacrocaudalis dorsalis medialis of a highly marbled, high Wagyu content (88%) steer M508 (wy63 ak25 dx13), showing variation of fiber size, with the presence of rounded fibers, internal nuclei, abundant perimysial connective tissue, and considerable adipose tissue. Formalin-fixed H & E, MSA MB 1100, DOF 471. CYO lab number Ch18/110G. See also ***Figure 1*** *for macroscopic comparison.*

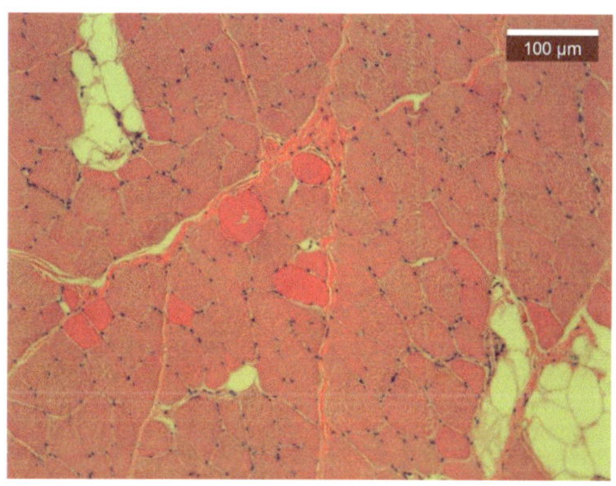

Figure 6.
Histological section of Sacrocaudalis dorsalis medialis of a highly marbled, high Wagyu content (75%) heifer M621 (wy75 dx25). Field selected to show eosinophilic rounded fibers of variable size, with abundant perimysial connective tissue in their proximity. Formalin-fixed H & E, MSA MB 820, DOF 471. CYO lab number Ch18/109Y. See also ***Figure 2*** *for macroscopic features such as coarse marbling.*

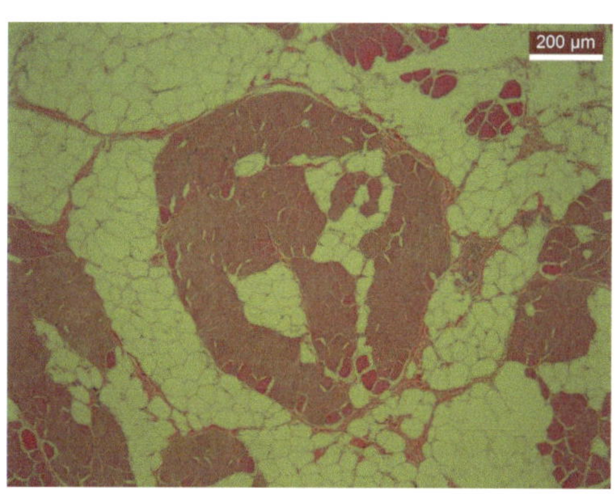

Figure 7.
Histological section of Sacrocaudalis dorsalis medialis of a highly marbled, high Wagyu content steer (88%) (wy63 ak25 dx13), showing aggressive adipose invasion, with abundant perimysial connective tissue and the generation of island-like areas of fibers with evident architectural changes including shrinkage of fibers as the front advances. Formalin-fixed H & E, MSA MB 1100, DOF 471. CYO lab number Ch18/110G. See also ***Figures 1, 4,*** *and* ***5****.*

In some fields, there are collections of nuclei including intracytoplasmic (**Figure 8**).

These observations have led us to the conclusion that the extent and type of marbling is a function of the aggressive extension of the advancing adipocytes with secondary loss of myocytes.

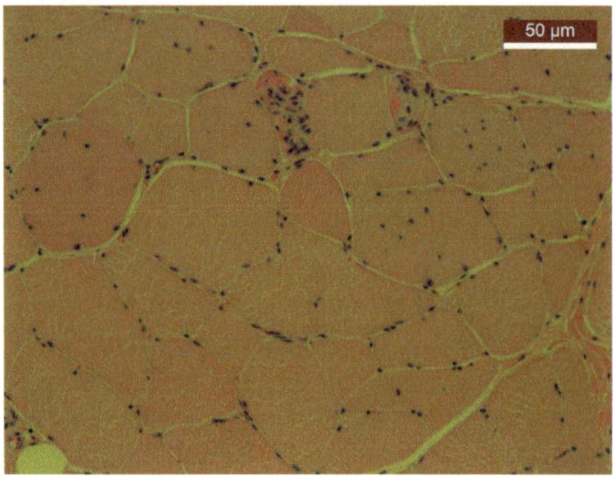

Figure 8.
Histological section of Sacrocaudalis dorsalis medialis of a highly marbled, high Wagyu content steer (63%), M129 (wy63 dx13). Higher power selected to illustrate variability of fiber size, affinity for eosin, and the presence of intracytoplasmatic and interstitial nuclei. Formalin-fixed H & E, MSA MB 880, DOF 481. CYO lab number Ch18/135Z.

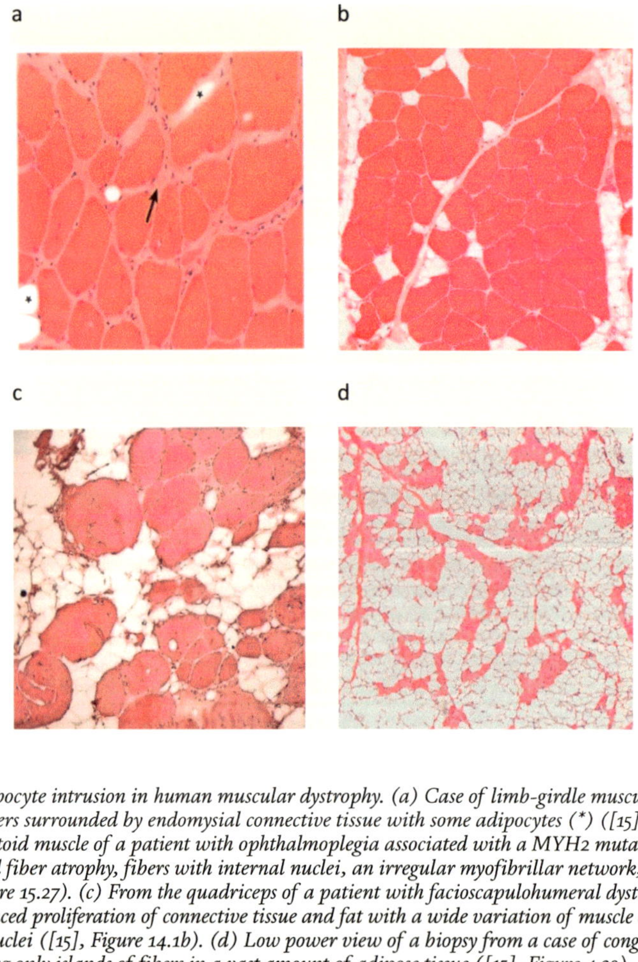

Figure 9.
Examples of adipocyte intrusion in human muscular dystrophy. (a) Case of limb-girdle muscular dystrophy showing most fibers surrounded by endomysial connective tissue with some adipocytes (*) ([15], Figure 11.4b). (b) From the deltoid muscle of a patient with ophthalmoplegia associated with a MYH2 mutation showing fatty infiltration, mild fiber atrophy, fibers with internal nuclei, an irregular myofibrillar network, and lobulated fibers ([15], Figure 15.27). (c) From the quadriceps of a patient with facioscapulohumeral dystrophy at 42 years showing pronounced proliferation of connective tissue and fat with a wide variation of muscle cell size and many internal nuclei ([15], Figure 14.1b). (d) Low power view of a biopsy from a case of congenital muscular dystrophy showing only islands of fibers in a vast amount of adipose tissue ([15], Figure 4.30).

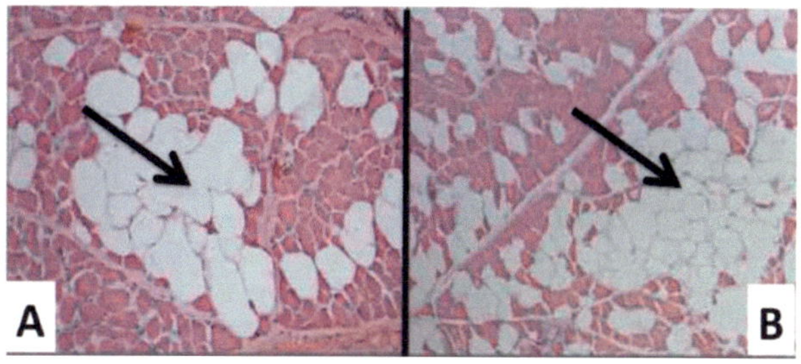

Figure 10.
Muscle samples taken from carcasses where steatosis was observed macroscopically at slaughter. Fat infiltration occurs within the muscle fascicle, there are few adipocytes within the perimysium. Used with permission from [17].

Some forms of human dystrophy have very similar histopathology, for example, congenital myopathies as illustrated by Dubowitz et al. [15] and reproduced here in **Figure 9**.

As in human dystrophies, there can be different degrees depending upon the muscle group and the field selected. Here, we focus on *Sacrocaudalis dorsalis medialis*, because it is convenient to biopsy, whereas the loin can only be accessed readily post-mortem.

Accordingly, it will be possible to undertake detailed time course studies so as to monitor sequential changes and eventually responses to therapy. Future studies should also address bovine steatosis. The pathology [16, 17] is different from marbling. Adipocytes occur within rather than around fascicles (**Figure 10**) suggesting that the process may be a function of differentiation of stem cells, rather than invasion [1].

7. Conclusion

In spite of similarities in pathology and genomics, there is more to learn before precise translation is possible. However, there are strong indications that such approaches could have important implications for human dystrophies and other muscle diseases. Moreover, a better understanding of the control factors and signals responsible for determining the relative proportions of muscle and adipose tissue in bovine muscles, and how they are coordinated, is fundamental and will be crucial to understanding more fully the significance of adipose tissue replacement in human dystrophies and to developing new therapeutic strategies for these diseases.

Acknowledgements

This research was supported by the CY O'Connor ERADE Village Foundation as publication number MS1803. The authors **acknowledge the earlier contributions of J F Williamson and** would like to thank JR Dawkins and Melaleuka Stud for access to the cattle used in this study.

Conflict of interest

Collectively, the authors associated with the CY O'Connor ERADE Village Foundation have an interest in the work described in this manuscript as it forms part of the foundation's intellectual property.

Author details

Jose L. Valenzuela[1,2], Sally S. Lloyd[1,2], Edward J. Steele[1,3], Francis L. Mastaglia[4] and Roger L. Dawkins[1,2*]

1 CY O'Connor ERADE Village Foundation, North Dandalup, Australia

2 Centre for Innovation in Agriculture, Murdoch University, Murdoch, Australia

3 Melville Analytics Pty Ltd, Melbourne, VIC, Australia

4 Queen Elizabeth II Medical Centre, Perron Institute for Neurological and Translational Science, Nedlands, WA, Australia

*Address all correspondence to: rldawkins@cyo.edu.au

References

[1] Harper GS, Pethick DW. How might marbling begin? Australian Journal of Experimental Agriculture. 2004;**44**:653-662

[2] Tan P, Allen JG, Wilton SD, et al. A splice-site mutation causing ovine McArdle's disease. Neuromuscular Disorders. 1997;7:336-342

[3] Ferreiro A, Ceuterick-De Groote C, Marks JJ, et al. Desmin-related myopathy with Mallory body-like inclusions is caused by mutations of the Selenoprotein N gene. Annals of Neurology. 2004;**55**:676-686

[4] Kakulas BA. Regeneration of skeletal muscle in the Rottnest quokka. The Australian Journal of Experimental Biology and Medical Science. 1966;**44**:673-688

[5] Williamson JF, Steele EJ, Lester S, et al. Genomic evolution in domestic cattle: Ancestral haplotypes and healthy beef. Genomics. 2011;**97**:304-312

[6] Dawkins RL, Leelayuwat C, Gaudieri S, et al. Genomics of the major histocompatibility complex: Haplotypes, duplication, retroviruses and disease. Immunological Reviews. 1999;**167**:275-304

[7] Aly TA, Eller E, Ide A, et al. Multi-SNP analysis of MHC region: Remarkable conservation of HLA-A1-B8-DR3 haplotype. Diabetes. 2006;**55**:1265-1269

[8] Lloyd SS, Steele EJ, Dawkins RL. Analysis of haplotype sequences. In: Kulski JK, editor. Next Generation Sequencing-Advances, Applications and Challenges. Rijeka, Croatia: InTech; 2016. pp. 345-368

[9] Traherne JA, Horton R, Roberts AN, et al. Genetic analysis of completely sequenced disease-associated MHC haplotypes identifies shuffling of segments in recent human history. PLoS Genetics. 2006;**2**:81-92

[10] Alper CA, Larsen CE, Dubey DP, et al. The haplotype structure of the human major histocompatibility complex. Human Immunology. 2006;**67**:73-84

[11] Dawkins RL, Willamson JF, Lester S, et al. Mutation versus polymorphism in evolution. Genomics. 2013;**101**:211-212

[12] Lloyd SS, Valenzuela JL, Steele EJ, et al. Genetics of marbling in Wagyu revealed by the melting temperature of intramuscular and subcutaneous lipids. International Journal of Food Science. 2017. Article ID 3948408, 6 pages

[13] Lloyd SS, Steele EJ, Valenzuela JL, et al. Haplotypes for type, degree and rate of marbling in cattle are syntenic with human muscular dystrophy. International Journal of Genomics. 2017;**2017**. Article ID 6532837, 14 pages

[14] Valenzuela JL, Lloyd SS, Rebhan H, et al. Monitoring marbling by histology and melting temperature. Pending Publ

[15] Dubowitz V, Sewry CA, Oldfors A, et al. Muscle Biopsy: A Practical Approach. Philadelphia: Saunders Ltd., 2013

[16] Peletto S, Strillacci MG, Capucchio MT, et al. Genetic basis of Lipomatous myopathy in Piedmontese beef cattle. Livestock Science. 2017;**206**:9-16

[17] Biasibetti E, Amedeo S, Brugiapaglia A, et al. Lipomatous muscular dystrophy' of Piedmontese cattle. Animal. 2012;**6**:1839-1847

[18] Tajsharghi H, Hammans S, Lindberg C, et al. Recessive myosin myopathy with external ophthalmoplegia associated with MYH2 mutations.

European Journal of Human Genetics. 2014;**22**:801-808

[19] Lim KS, Lee SH, Lee EA, et al. Effects of intergenic single nucleotide polymorphisms in the fast myosin heavy chain cluster on muscle fiber characteristics and meat quality in Berkshire pigs. Meat Science. Epub ahead of print 2015. DOI: 10.1016/j.meatsci.2015.07.025

[20] Nobbio L, Visigalli D, Radice D, et al. PMP22 messenger RNA levels in skin biopsies: Testing the effectiveness of a Charcot-Marie-Tooth 1A biomarker. Brain. 2014;**137**:1614-1620

[21] Iwata Y, Katanosaka Y, Arai Y, et al. Dominant-negative inhibition of Ca2+ influx via TRPV2 ameliorates muscular dystrophy in animal models. Human Molecular Genetics. 2009;**18**:824-834

[22] Lloyd DJ, Trembath RC, Shackleton S. A novel interaction between lamin A and SREBP1: Implications for partial lipodystrophy and other laminopathies. Human Molecular Genetics. 2002;**11**: 769-778

[23] Hoashi S, Ashida N, Ohsaki H, et al. Genotype of bovine sterol regulatory element binding protein-1 (SREBP-1) is associated with fatty acid composition in Japanese Black cattle. Mammalian Genome. 2007;**18**:880-886

[24] Surks HK, Riddick N, Ohtani K-I. M-RIP targets myosin phosphatase to stress fibers to regulate myosin light chain phosphorylation in vascular smooth muscle cells. Journal of Biological Chemistry. Epub ahead of print 2005. DOI: 10.1074/jbc.M506863200

[25] Dawkins RL, Millman JA, Willamson JF, et al. US9181585B2. pdf. US 9,181,585 B2, United States of America; 2015

[26] Trabelsi M, Kavian N, Daoud F, et al. Revised spectrum of mutations in sarcoglycanopathies. European Journal of Human Genetics. 2008;**16**:793-803

[27] Moreira ES, Wiltshire TJ, Faulkner G, et al. Limb-girdle muscular dystrophy type 2G is caused by mutations in the gene encoding the sarcomeric protein telethonin. Nature Genetics. 2000;**24**:163-166

[28] Cheong HS, Yoon D, Kim LH, et al. Titin-cap (TCAP) polymorphisms associated with marbling score of beef. Meat Science. 2007;**77**:257-263

[29] Hayashi YK, Matsuda C, Ogawa M, et al. Human PTRF mutations cause secondary deficiency of caveolins resulting in muscular dystrophy with generalized lipodystrophy. Journal of Clinical Investigation. 2009;**119**:2623-2633

[30] Grumati P, Coletto L, Sabatelli P, et al. Autophagy is defective in collagen VI muscular dystrophies, and its reactivation rescues myofiber degeneration. Nature Medicine 2010;**16**:1313-1320

[31] García-Macia M, Sierra V, Palanca A, et al. Autophagy during beef aging. Autophagy. Epub ahead of print 2014. DOI: 10.4161/auto.26659

[32] Ardiyanti A, Oki Y, Suda Y, et al. Effects of GH gene polymorphism and sex on carcass traits and fatty acid compositions in Japanese Black cattle. Journal of Animal Science. 2009;**80**:62-69

[33] Bhuiyan MSA, Kim YK, Kim HJ, et al. Genome-wide association study and prediction of genomic breeding values for fatty-acid composition in Korean Hanwoo cattle using a high-density single-nucleotide polymorphism array1. Journal of Animal Science. 2018;**96**:4063-4075

[34] Uemoto Y, Abe T, Tameoka N, et al. Whole-genome association study for

fatty acid composition of oleic acid in Japanese Black cattle. Animal Genetics. 2011;**42**:141-148

[35] Schuelke M, Wagner KR, Stolz LE, et al. Myostatin mutation associated with gross muscle hypertrophy in a child. The New England Journal of Medicine. 2004;**350**:2682-2688

[36] Wiener P, Woolliams JA, Frank-Lawale A, et al. The effects of a mutation in the myostatin gene on meat and carcass quality. Meat Science. Epub ahead of print 2009. DOI: 10.1016/j.meatsci.2009.04.010

[37] Barendse W, Harrison BE, Bunch RJ, et al. Variation at the Calpain 3 gene is associated with meat tenderness in zebu and composite breeds of cattle. BMC Genetics. Epub ahead of print 2008. DOI: 10.1186/1471-2156-9-41

[38] Casas E, White SN, Riley DG, et al. Assessment of single nucleotide polymorphisms in genes residing on chromosomes 14 and 29 for association with carcass composition traits in Bos indicus cattle. Journal of Animal Science. 2005;**83**:13-19

[39] Adoligbe CLZ, Farougou S. Functional analysis and association studies of bovine MYOT gene with meat quality. Journal of Animal Science. 2016;**94**:59-60